10th Anniversary of *Children*: Feature Papers in Neonatology

10th Anniversary of *Children*: Feature Papers in Neonatology

Guest Editor

Karel Allegaert

MDPI

Basel • Beijing • Wuhan • Barcelona • Belgrade • Novi Sad • Cluj • Manchester

Guest Editor
Karel Allegaert
Department of Development
and Regeneration
KU Leuven
Leuven
Belgium

Editorial Office
MDPI AG
Grosspeteranlage 5
4052 Basel, Switzerland

This is a reprint of the Special Issue, published open access by the journal *Children* (ISSN 2227-9067), freely accessible at: https://www.mdpi.com/journal/children/special_issues/YA87NQO0QJ.

For citation purposes, cite each article independently as indicated on the article page online and as indicated below:

Lastname, A.A.; Lastname, B.B. Article Title. *Journal Name* **Year**, *Volume Number*, Page Range.

ISBN 978-3-7258-4261-2 (Hbk)
ISBN 978-3-7258-4262-9 (PDF)
https://doi.org/10.3390/books978-3-7258-4262-9

Contents

children

MDPI

Editorial

The Special Issue on Neonatology for the 10th Anniversary of *Children*: From Preclinical Findings to Bringing Families to the Centre of Contemporary Neonatal Care

Karel Allegaert [1,2,3]

[1] Department of Pharmaceutical and Pharmacological Sciences, KU Leuven, 3000 Leuven, Belgium; karel.allegaert@kuleuven.be
[2] Department of Development and Regeneration, KU Leuven, 3000 Leuven, Belgium
[3] Department of Hospital Pharmacy, Erasmus MC, 3015 GD Rotterdam, The Netherlands

1. Introduction

Neonatology is a specialized branch of medicine, focussed on the care of newborns, either related to preterm birth or other medical conditions like sepsis, asphyxia, or congenital malformations. In the 1960s, specialized neonatal intensive care units (NICU) emerged, transforming the care landscape for newborns, informed by other disciplines, and evolving from eminence-based practices to more evidence-based approaches [1].

Weighted to other disciplines, this means that our discipline is still rather young; therefore, there is still much to investigate, as reflected in the diversity of topics covered in the current Special Issue [1]. In addition, the creation of NICUs also resulted in a more robust ecosystem, with a higher degree of confidence and opportunities to shift to the treatment of neonates with more complex care demands, like micro-preemies, or complex cardiac malformations or genetic syndromes. Treatment modalities changed, from delivery room management to care bundle concepts (respiratory, neurological, nutritional, pharmacological, and family-centred care), as have the outcomes of preterm neonates or neonates with specific conditions [2,3]. Related to prevention, screening and treatment have evolved significantly over the last decade, improving outcomes. Prevention and screening strategies have been developed and implemented for prenatal screening, dry blood spots, cardiac screening, and hearing screening [4].

This diversity is also reflected in the topics covered in this Special Issue, ranging from preclinical (murine model, human milk fat composition) and epidemiology (impact of race on outcome, impact of fetal growth restriction on behavioural outcome), to guidelines (oxygenation monitoring, hypoglycemia) and several papers on family-centred care and parent-related impact (impact of family-centred and developmental care on outcome, relevance of the family context, post-discharge impact of parent support), ending with two papers on screening-related practices (mother's knowledge on dried blood spot screening, usefulness of polymorphism screening for neonatal bilirubinaemia management).

2. Overview of the Published Articles

2.1. Pre-Clinical

In a preclinical murine bronchopulmonary dysplasia model (BPD), Chen et al. observed that neonatal hyperoxia exposure caused an arrest of lung development, as well as an obstacle to the myelination process in the white matter of the immature brain, with a decline in myeline basic protein in the generation period of myelin and persistent as-

 https://doi.org/10.3390/children12050622

trogliosis (contribution 1). This informs us that BPD is a systemic disease, not limited to the pulmonary system.

The impact of human milk fatty acid composition on growth velocity in preterm infants was reported by Ahmed et al. In essence, and based on 15 mother–infant dyads, the growth velocity increased with the decrement in C16 and increment in C20:2n6, while the lipid profile of preterm human milk was found to be low for some essential fatty acids, which may affect the quality of preterm infants' nutrition (contribution 2). Interestingly, there is a link between both findings, as the lipid profile is also crucial to ensure myelination.

2.2. Epidemiology

The progress mentioned in the introduction is most clearly reflected in the data on mortality. Qattea et al. hereby described that there has been a significant decrease in mortality in black and white populations in the last two decades in the United States (contribution 3). However, when stratifying the population by many significant epidemiologic and hospital factors, the mortality remained consistently higher in black populations throughout the study years.

In a Spanish cohort of 70 former fetal growth-restriction cases, behavioural performance was assessed at the age of 6 years by Benitez Marin et al. Higher behavioural disability rates were observed, providing additional evidence on the negative relationship between the birth weight percentile and the total behavioural scale score (contribution 4). Both papers inform us on the clinical relevance of specific covariates that determine short- or long-term outcome of former NICU graduates.

2.3. Guideline Adherence

European guidelines recommend the use of pulse oximetry (PO) during newborn resuscitation, especially when there is a need for positive pressure ventilation or supplemental oxygen. Kolstad et al. therefore evaluated these practices based on video recordings in 230 ventilated newborns at delivery. In total, 97% of resuscitated newborns had PO applied, in line with resuscitation guidelines. However, the proportion of time with a useful PO signal during ventilation and during the first 10 minutes on the resuscitation table was only 5% and 35%, respectively (contribution 5).

Neonatal hypoglycemia remains an issue of debate as it is a preventable cause of brain injury and neurodevelopmental impairment. Unfortunately, Giouleka et al. had to conclude that—after a comprehensive review on the guidelines—there is still no clear definition, nor consistent treatment policy. Thus, the establishment of specific diagnostic criteria and uniform protocols for the management of this common biochemical disorder is of paramount importance as it may allow early identification of infants at risk and the establishment of effective preventive measures or treatments to improvement outcomes (contribution 6).

Both papers are quite illustrative of the logistics related to and the complexity of either implementing what is already known (the pulse oximetry measurement during neonatal ventilation), while the paper on neonatal hypoglycemia reinforms us on the many known unknows in this field.

2.4. Parents Matter, Bringing Families to the Centre of Contemporary Neonatal Care

Based on a pre-post design in 200 high-risk preterm neonates with family-centred care and developmental care in the intervention group, Alsadaan et al. reported that family centred care and developmental care in the intervention group were associated with improved cognitive, motor, and language scores, as well as with a shorter length of stay (contribution 7).

In a qualitative descriptive study on parent and NICU clinician experiences and perspectives, Dahan et al. concluded that their study highlights how the quality of care is positively impacted by clinicians' appreciation of the family context and the complex relationship between a large multidisciplinary interprofessional team and the family in an intensive care unit, while also highlighting the difficulties in its practical application (contribution 8).

Post discharge, Munoz et al. observed that parent support (supportive presence and quality of assistance during a complex problem-solving task) had the greatest impact on high-birth risk ($\leq$27 gestational weeks) toddler brain development (frontal lobe grey matter volume, emotion regulation); thus, early parent interventions may normalize preterm child neurodevelopment and have lasting impacts (contribution 9).

All papers clearly illustrate and stress that families should be at the centre of contemporary neonatal care, and that this is not limited to during the neonatal stay but clearly extends to the impact and outcome after discharge.

2.5. Screening/Prevention

Di Gangi et al. explored what mothers know about newborn bloodspot screening and the source they use to acquire this knowledge in a Flemish representative sample of 200 subjects and hereby concluded that the consent practices and knowledge level was reasonably good, the information leaflets were perceived to be supporting, while key health care providers were midwives and nurses (contribution 10).

In a well conducted study, Riskin et al. reported that both the genetics of glucose-6-phosphate-dehydrogenase (G6PD) and Uridine Diphosphate Glucuronosyl Transferase 1A1 (UGT1A1) were associated with higher risks of developing clinically relevant neonatal hyperbilirubinemia. The results of this study highlight the possibility for future implementation of molecular genetic screening to identify infants at specific increased risk for significant neonatal hyperbilirubinemia (contribution 11).

A lot of new ideas or concepts have emerged in the field of neonatal newborn bloodspot screening, including a shift towards whole genome screening concepts. The paper on bilirubin-related polymorphisms illustrates one potential useful application, while Di Gangi informs us that we should not forget effective communication with parents and healthcare providers to ensure appropriate consent practices, knowledge level, and overall confidence in these practices.

3. Conclusions

In conclusion, the diversity of topics and aspects covered reflect the diversity of research lines needed to make progress, unveil knowledge gaps, share practices, and shift further towards a more evidence-based approach to ensure further improvements in outcomes.

Funding: This research received no external funding.

Conflicts of Interest: The author declare no conflicts of interest.

List of Contributions:

1. Chen, W.; Wang, R.; Chen, C. Cerebral Myelination in a Bronchopulmonary Dysplasia Murine Model. *Children* **2023**, *10*, 1321. https://doi.org/10.3390/children10081321.
2. Ahmed, B.; Freije, A.; Omran, A.; Rondanelli, M.; Marino, M.; Perna, S. Human Milk Fatty Acid Composition and Its Effect on Preterm Infants' Growth Velocity. *Children* **2023**, *10*, 939. https://doi.org/10.3390/children10060939.
3. Qattea, I.; Burdjalov, M.; Quatei, A.; Agha, K.T.; Kteish, R.; Aly, H. Disparities in Neonatal Mortalities in the United States. *Children* **2023**, *10*, 1386. https://doi.org/10.3390/children10081386.

4. Benítez Marín, M.J.; Blasco Alonso, M.; González Mesa, E. Prenatal Predictors of Neurobehavioral Outcome in Children with Fetal Growth Restriction at 6 Years of Age: A Retrospective Cohort Study. *Children* **2023**, *10*, 997. https://doi.org/10.3390/children10060997.
5. Kolstad, V.; Pike, H.; Eilevstjønn, J.; Buskov, F.; Ersdal, H.; Rettedal, S. Use of Pulse Oximetry during Resuscitation of 230 Newborns—A Video Analysis. *Children* **2023**, *10*, 1124. https://doi.org/10.3390/children10071124.
6. Giouleka, S.; Gkiouleka, M.; Tsakiridis, I.; Daniilidou, A.; Mamopoulos, A.; Athanasiadis, A.; Dagklis, T. Diagnosis and Management of Neonatal Hypoglycemia: A Comprehensive Review of Guidelines. *Children* **2023**, *10*, 1220. https://doi.org/10.3390/children10071220.
7. Alsadaan, N.; Ramadan, O.M.E.; Alqahtani, M.; Shaban, M.; Elsharkawy, N.B.; Abdelaziz, E.M.; Ali, S.I. Impacts of Integrating Family-Centered Care and Developmental Care Principles on Neonatal Neurodevelopmental Outcomes among High-Risk Neonates. *Children* **2023**, *10*, 1751. https://doi.org/10.3390/children10111751.
8. Dahan, M.; Rotteau, L.; Higazi, S.; Kwayke, O.; Lai, G.; Moulsdale, W.; Sampson, L.; Stannard, J.; Church, P.T.; O'Brien, K. Understanding the Family Context: A Qualitative Descriptive Study of Parent and NICU Clinician Experiences and Perspectives. *Children* **2023**, *10*, 896. https://doi.org/10.3390/children10050896.
9. Muñoz, J.S.; Giles, M.E.; Vaughn, K.A.; Wang, Y.; Landry, S.H.; Bick, J.R.; DeMaster, D.M. Parenting Influences on Frontal Lobe Gray Matter and Preterm Toddlers' Problem-Solving Skills. *Children* **2024**, *11*, 206. https://doi.org/10.3390/children11020206.
10. di Gangi, C.; Hermans, M.; Rayyan, M.; Eyskens, F.; Allegaert, K. What Mothers Know about Newborn Bloodspot Screening and the Sources They Use to Acquire This Knowledge: A Pilot Study in Flanders. *Children* **2023**, *10*, 1567. https://doi.org/10.3390/children10091567.
11. Riskin, A.; Bravdo, Y.; Habib, C.; Maor, I.; Mousa, J.; Shahbarat, S.; Shahak, E.; Shalata, A. The Genetics of Glucose-6-Phosphate-Dehydrogenase (G6PD) and Uridine Diphosphate Glucuronosyl Transferase 1A1 (UGT1A1) Promoter Gene Polymorphism in Relation to Quantitative Biochemical G6PD Activity Measurement and Neonatal Hyperbilirubinemia. *Children* **2023**, *10*, 1172. https://doi.org/10.3390/children10071172.

References

1. Oei, J.L.; Martin, R.J. Therapeutic drift in newborn, care- an evaluation of common practices with little or no evidence. *Sem. Fetal Neonatal Med.* **2021**, *26*, 101226. [CrossRef] [PubMed]
2. Amuji, N.; Rao, S.A.; Nagaraju, P.Y.; Suresh, K.G.; Steven, S.; Shekharappa, C.B. Improving the quality of care for preterm infants in the golden hour. *BMJ Open Qual.* **2025**, *14*, e002277. [CrossRef] [PubMed]
3. Mitra, S.; Dorling, J.; Johnston, B.C. Optimizing practice guidelines through incorporating patient and family values and preferences. *Sem. Fetal Neonatal Med.* **2021**, *26*, 101194. [CrossRef] [PubMed]
4. Bick, D.; Ahmed, A.; Deen, D.; Ferlini, A.; Garnier, N.; Kasperaviciute, D.; Leblond, M.; Pichini, A.; Rendon, A.; Satija, A.; et al. Newborn Screening by Genomic Sequencing: Opportunities and Challenges. *Int. J. Neonatal Screen.* **2022**, *8*, 40. [CrossRef] [PubMed]

children

MDPI

Review

Diagnosis and Management of Neonatal Hypoglycemia: A Comprehensive Review of Guidelines

Sonia Giouleka [1], Maria Gkiouleka [2], Ioannis Tsakiridis [1,*], Anastasia Daniilidou [1], Apostolos Mamopoulos [1], Apostolos Athanasiadis [1] and Themistoklis Dagklis [1]

[1] Third Department of Obstetrics and Gynecology, School of Medicine, Faculty of Health Sciences, Aristotle University of Thessaloniki, Konstantinoupoleos 49, 54642 Thessaloniki, Greece; soniagiouleka@outlook.com (S.G.); daniilidouanastasia@gmail.com (A.D.); amamop@auth.gr (A.M.); apostolos3435@gmail.com (A.A.); tdagklis@gmail.com (T.D.)

[2] University College London Hospital, University College London Medical School, 250 Euston Road, London NW1 2PG, UK; mariagkiouleka@outlook.com

* Correspondence: iotsakir@gmail.com; Tel.: +30-2313312120; Fax: +30-2310-992950

Abstract: Hypoglycemia represents one of the most frequent metabolic disturbances of the neonate, associated with increased morbidity and mortality, especially if left untreated or diagnosed after the establishment of brain damage. The aim of this study was to review and compare the recommendations from the most recently published influential guidelines on the diagnosis, screening, prevention and management of this common neonatal complication. Therefore, a descriptive review of the guidelines from the American Academy of Pediatrics (AAP), the British Association of Perinatal Medicine (BAPM), the European Foundation for the Care of the Newborn Infants (EFCNI), the Queensland Clinical Guidelines-Australia (AUS), the Canadian Pediatric Society (CPS) and the Pediatric Endocrine Society (PES) on neonatal hypoglycemia was carried out. There is a consensus among the reviewed guidelines on the risk factors, the clinical signs and symptoms of NH, and the main preventive strategies. Additionally, the importance of early recognition of at-risk infants, timely identification of NH and prompt initiation of treatment in optimizing the outcomes of hypoglycemic neonates are universally highlighted. All medical societies, except PES, recommend screening for NH in asymptomatic high-risk and symptomatic newborn infants, but they do not provide consistent screening approaches. Moreover, the reviewed guidelines point out that the diagnosis of NH should be confirmed by laboratory methods of BGL measurement, although treatment should not be delayed until the results become available. The definition of NH lacks uniformity and it is generally agreed that a single BG value cannot accurately define this clinical entity. Therefore, all medical societies support the use of operational thresholds for the management of NH, although discrepancies exist regarding the recommended cut-off values, the optimal treatment and surveillance strategies of both symptomatic and asymptomatic hypoglycemic neonates as well as the treatment targets. Over the past several decades, NH has remained an issue of keen debate as it is a preventable cause of brain injury and neurodevelopmental impairment; however, there is no clear definition or consistent treatment policies. Thus, the establishment of specific diagnostic criteria and uniform protocols for the management of this common biochemical disorder is of paramount importance as it will hopefully allow for the early identification of infants at risk, the establishment of efficient preventive measures, the optimal treatment in the first hours of a neonate's life and, subsequently, the improvement of neonatal outcomes.

Keywords: neonatal hypoglycemia; blood glucose levels; plasma glucose; glucose; dextrose; diagnosis; definition; operational threshold; risk factors; clinical signs; screening; management; guidelines; comparison

1. Introduction

Neonatal hypoglycemia (NH) is the most common neonatal metabolic disturbance [1] and constitutes a leading cause of term admission to neonatal units worldwide [2]. Its incidence is estimated to be 5–15% in otherwise healthy neonates [3,4]. The definition of clinically significant hypoglycemia remains one of the most controversial issues in contemporary neonatology, as blood glucose (BG) concentration is not routinely measured in healthy asymptomatic infants who may experience transient hypoglycemia as part of their normal adaptation to extrauterine life [5]. Thus, the normal range of blood glucose levels (BGL) in the first 48 h of life is yet to be determined [1].

Delayed diagnosis, as well as the suboptimal management of NH, is associated with adverse short- and long-term sequelae in the offspring; acute brain injury, visual-motor impairment, executive dysfunction and neurodevelopmental impairment have been reported [6–8]. It is worth noting that despite the fact that several studies and clinical trials have attempted to identify the BGL considered to be safe and to provide a valid estimate of the effect of neonatal hypoglycemia on neurodevelopment [9], evidence from the current literature does not support a specific concentration of BG that can potentially result in acute or chronic irreversible neurologic damage and neither the duration nor the severity of NH can accurately predict permanent neurological damage [6].

Although occasions where NH is severe enough to cause long-term neurodevelopmental harm with subsequent significant costs for the family, the patients and the health systems are rare [10], clinicians should implement practices to prevent harm stemming from failure to recognize or treat NH whilst eliminating unnecessary interventions and admissions to neonatal units and, therefore, avoiding the pointless separation between the mother and the neonate. To date, there is insufficient and inconclusive evidence regarding the definition and treatment protocols of NH, leading to significant discrepancies in the existing guidelines. Thus, the development of international evidence-based algorithms for the early identification, the effective prevention and the successful management of clinically significant low BGL seems to be of insurmountable importance and will hopefully drive favorable neonatal outcomes.

The aim of this descriptive review was to synthesize and compare recommendations from influential guidelines on the diagnosis and management of neonatal hypoglycemia.

2. Evidence Acquisition

The most recently published guidelines by influential medical societies on NH were retrieved and a descriptive review was conducted. In particular, six guidelines were identified from: the American Academy of Pediatrics (AAP 2011) [11], the British Association of Perinatal Medicine (BAPM 2017) [12], the European Foundation for the Care of the Newborn Infants (EFCNI 2018) [13], the Queensland Clinical Guidelines-Australia (AUS 2019) [14], the Canadian Pediatric Society (CPS 2020) [15] and the Pediatric Endocrine Society (PES 2015) [16].

An overview of recommendations is presented in Table 1 (risk factors and clinical signs of NH) and Table 2 (screening, diagnosis and management of NH), respectively. Of note, five of the reviewed guidelines focus mostly on the transitional NH in the immediate postnatal period; however, the recommendations made by PES mainly address the subject of persistent NH, including the diagnosis and management of disorders causing recurrent or prolonged hypoglycemia that persists or occurs beyond the first 72 h of life.

Table 1. Risk factors and clinical signs of neonatal hypoglycemia.

	AAP	BAPM	EFCNI	AUS	CPS	PES
Country	United States	United Kingdom	Europe	Australia	Canada	International
Issued	March 2011	April 2017	November 2018	September 2019	December 2020	August 2015
Title	Clinical Report—Postnatal Glucose Homeostasis in Late-Preterm and Term Infants	Identification and Management of Neonatal Hypoglycemia in the Full Term Infant	Hypoglycemia in at-risk term infants	Hypoglycemia–newborn	The screening and management of newborns at risk for low blood glucose	Recommendations from the Pediatric Endocrine Society for Evaluation and Management of Persistent Hypoglycemia in Neonates, Infants and Children
Pages	7	35	8	38	17	8
References	31	81	24	75	75	39
Risk factors	SGA, LGA, maternal diabetes, late prematurity	FGR, maternal diabetes, maternal beta-blockers in 3rd trim +/− at delivery), moderate to severe perinatal hypoxia-ischemia, suspected/confirmed early onset sepsis, pituitary/adrenal insufficiency, inborn errors of metabolism, hyperinsulinism, family history of 1st degree relative with a heritable hypoglycemic disorder.	FGR, maternal diabetes, asphyxia, maternal beta-blockers, sepsis, hemolytic disease, specific inborn errors of metabolism, congenital disorders that prevent infants from mounting an adequate counter-regulatory metabolic and endocrine response.	FGR, LGA, macrosomia, maternal medication, maternal diabetes, hyperinsulinemia, family history of genetic form of hypoglycemia or congenital hyper-insulinemic or endocrine disorder, sibling or parent with MCADD, PE/eclampsia or GH or other placental insufficiency, intrapartum IV glucose > 20 g/h, neonate's T < 36.5 °C, perinatal asphyxia, PTL or postmature, neonate with seizures, delayed/inadequate feeding, IV therapy–abrupt cessation or rapid weaning of glucose, meconium aspiration, polycythemia, hypothyroidism, severe hepatic dysfunction, erythroblastosis, inborn errors of metabolism.	SGA, FGR, LGA, maternal diabetes, prematurity maternal labetalol use, late exposure to antenatal steroids, perinatal asphyxia, metabolic conditions, syndromes associated with hypoglycemia.	FGR, LGA, SGA, perinatal stress/asphyxia/ischemia, PE/eclampsia or GH, meconium aspiration, erythroblastosis, polycythemia, hypothermia PTL or postmature delivery, maternal diabetes, family history of a genetic form of hypoglycemia, congenital syndromes, abnormal physical features (midline facial malformation, microphallus).

Table 1. *Cont.*

	AAP	BAPM	EFCNI	AUS	CPS	PES
Clinical signs of NH	Jitteriness, cyanosis, seizures, apneic episodes, tachypnea, weak or high-pitched cry, floppiness or lethargy, poor feeding, eye-rolling. Coma and seizures if prolonged and repetitive NH.	Perinatal acidosis, T < 36.5 °C, early onset sepsis, cyanosis, apnea, altered level of consciousness, seizures, hypotonia, lethargy, high-pitched cry, abnormal feeding especially after a period of feeding well, jitteriness.	Abnormal feeding	Apnea, bradycardia, cyanosis, tachypnea, hypothermia, jitteriness, persistent tremor, irregular breathing, sweating, irritability, pallor, poor feeding, hypotonia, abnormal cry, seizures, changes in level of consciousness–stupor, coma, lethargy, apathy.	Jitteriness or tremors, cyanosis, convulsions, intermittent apneic spells or tachypnea, weak or high-pitched crying, limpness or lethargy, abnormal feeding, eye-rolling, sweating, sudden pallor, hypothermia, cardiac arrest and failure.	Palpitations, tremor, anxiety, sweating, hunger, paresthesia, confusion, coma and seizures.

LGA: large-for-gestational-age; SGA: small-for-gestational-age; FGR: fetal growth restriction; MCADD: medium chain acyl-CoA dehydrogenase deficiency; PE: preeclampsia; GH: gestational hypertension; T: temperature; PTL: preterm labor; IV: intravenous; NH: neonatal hypoglycemia.

Table 2. Summary of recommendations on screening, diagnosis and management of NH.

	AAP	BAPM	EFCNI	AUS	CPS	PES
Country	United States	United Kingdom	Europe	Australia	Canada	International
Issued	March 2011	April 2017	November 2018	September 2019	December 2020	August 2015
Title	Clinical Report—Postnatal Glucose Homeostasis in Late-Preterm and Term Infants	Identification and Management of Neonatal Hypoglycemia in the Full Term Infant	Hypoglycemia in at risk term infants	Hypoglycemia–newborn	The screening and management of newborns at risk for low blood glucose	Recommendations from the Pediatric Endocrine Society for Evaluation and Management of Persistent Hypoglycemia in Neonates, Infants and Children
Pages	7	35	8	38	17	8
References	31	81	24	75	75	39

Table 2. *Cont.*

	AAP	BAPM	EFCNI	AUS	CPS	PES
Screening for NH	Recommended in term infants with clinical signs or at risk. PG (within minutes, not hours) if clinical signs of low BGL. Frequency and duration individualized. At-risk infants should be fed by 1 h of age and screened 30 min later. After 24 h, repeat before feedings if PG remains <45 mg/dL.	Recommended if abnormal clinical signs, reluctant/non-effective feeding after a period of effective feeding, infants not effectively fed. Optimal time to measure BGL: prior to second feed (<4 h of delivery). If no feeding cues within 4 h, measure BG.	Recommended before the 2nd feed and no later than 4 h after birth in asymptomatic infants, or at any time if abnormal clinical signs.	Screening times: 1st BGL before 2nd feed and <3 h of age. 2nd BGL screen before 3rd feed and <6 h of age. If normal (≥2.6 mmol/L), screen before every 2nd feed–every 3–6 h pre-feed for 24 h.	Recommended for asymptomatic, at-risk infants at 2 h of age and 30 min post feed. When 2 consecutive samples are >2.6 mmol/L, continue monitoring pre-feed or every 3–6 h. Symptomatic and unwell infants require immediate glucose testing. Screen once or twice on day 2 when more than one PG < 2.6 mmol/L in the first 24 h.	Not discussed
Diagnosis-Operational Thresholds	PG concentration defining NH for all infants < 47 mg/dL. Operational thresholds: 25–40 mg/dL (1.4–2.2 mmol/L) in first 4 h, 35–45 mg/dL (1.9–2.5 mmol/L) from 4–24 h and 45 mg/dL (2.5 mmol/L) after 24 h of life.	BGL < 1.0 mmol/L at any time (severe hypoglycemia). A single BGL < 2.5 mmol/L if abnormal clinical signs. BGL < 2.0 mmol/L and remaining < 2.0 mmol/L at next measurement in at-risk baby, without clinical signs. Persistent hypoglycemia: ≥3 measurements <2.0 mmol/L in the first 48 h. Consider hyperinsulinism if BGL remain low (<2.0 mmol/L on ≥3 occasions in first 48 h), or if glucose dose > 8 mg/kg/min required. BGL threshold 3.0 mmol/L if suspected hyperinsulinism < 48 h after birth.	BGL < 1.0 mmol/L (18 mg/dL) associated with acute neurological dysfunction present the greatest risk of cerebral injury.	NH definition: symptomatic baby and/or BGL < 2.6 mmol/L. Severe hypoglycemia: BGL < 1.5 mmol/L. Prolonged hypoglycemia: >48 h. Recurrent hypoglycemia: ≥3 sequential episodes of BGL < 2.6 mmol/L.	Transitional hypoglycemia < 72 h post-birth: BGL < 2.6 mmol/L. Persistent hypoglycemia: BGL < 3.3 mmol/L > 72 h post-birth. Threshold BGL that requires action: 2.0 mmol/L.	Normal PG > 48 h: 70–100 mg/dL (3.9–5.5 mmol/L). Normal PG < 48: >55–65 mg/dL (3.0–3.6 mmol/L). In suspected congenital hypoglycemia disorder and older infants and children with a confirmed hypoglycemia disorder, treatment target recommended: PG > 70 mg/dL (3.9 mmol/L). For high-risk neonates without a suspected congenital hypoglycemia disorder, treatment target suggested: PG > 50 mg/dL (>2.8 mmol/L) < 48 h and >60 mg/dL (>3.3 mmol/L) > 48 h.

Table 2. *Cont.*

	AAP	BAPM	EFCNI	AUS	CPS	PES
Diagnostic methods	Laboratory enzymatic methods (Glucose oxidase, hexokinase or Dehydrogenase). Consider bedside reagent test-strip glucose analyzers (handheld reflectance colorimeter and electrode methods) if test performed carefully and clinician aware of their limited accuracy.	Ward-based blood gas biosensor (reference standard for measuring BG). Hand-held glucometers (prone to limited accuracy particularly in the range 0–2.0 mmol/L, -only use if ISO15197:2013 standard).	Ward-based blood gas biosensor (reference standard for measuring BG). Hand-held glucometers conforming to the ISO 15197:2013 standard (inaccurate particularly in the range 0–2.0 mmol/L).	Point of care glucometer with enzymatic methods (glucose oxidase or dehydrogenase). Otherwise, a calibrated non-enzymatic glucometer with electrochemical sensor validated for neonatal samples (may be unreliable at lower BGLs). If screening BGL < 2.6 mmol/L or borderline in a neonate at risk or with clinical signs of hypo-glycemia: Validate by diagnostic test using point of care analyzer, blood gas analyzer or laboratory specimen in fluoride oxalate tube.	While acute management can be initiated based on point-of-care samples to prevent delay, a diagnosis of persistent hypoglycemia should be confirmed by laboratory assays. Continuous glucose monitors (CGMs) of questionable accuracy.	Clinical laboratory method. Point-of-care meters: convenient screening method but with limited accuracy. Before establishing a diagnosis of NH, essential to confirm low PG by a clinical laboratory method.
Prevention	Not discussed	Keep neonate dried and warm with hat and blanket after birth. Skin-to-skin contact with the mother. Encourage early breast feeding within the 1st hour after birth. Not without meal for >3 h. Regular neonatal assessment when awake (color, tone, RR, HR, T, level of consciousness and signs of hypoglycemia).	Thermal care with skin-to-skin contact. Support breast feeding and discuss feeding cues. Early energy provision. Monitoring of BGL starting within the first hours of life.	Assess for RF. Keep baby warm and dried. Maintain T 36.5–37.5 °C. Early to skin contact. Initiate feeds within 30–60 min of birth. Feed at least three times hourly or more frequently. Formula feed if maternal choice or with consent if breast milk not available (at risk baby: 60–75 mL/kg/day as tolerated). If baby < 35 w admit to NICU. If clinical condition allows, early—frequent feeds.	Increase breastfeeding frequency. Supplement feeds with breast milk or breast milk substitute. Slow feeding with breast milk or formula using a pump rather than bolus feeding. Increase carbohydrate intake. Delay the first bath.	For disorders such as hyperinsulinism, aim to prevent recurrent hypoglycemia that increases the risk of subsequent, possibly unrecognized, hypoglycemic episodes.

Table 2. *Cont.*

	AAP	BAPM	EFCNI	AUS	CPS	PES
Management of asymptomatic NH	Asymptomatic at-risk infants should be fed by 1 h of age and screened 30 min later. If BGL < 25 mg/dL (<4 h of age) or <35 mg/dL (4–24 h of age), refeed and recheck BG 1 h later. Subsequent BGL < 25 mg/dL, or <35 mg/dL, respectively, after attempts to refeed, necessitate IV glucose treatment.	Neonates with pre-feed BG 1.0–1.9 mmol/L and no abnormal clinical signs or neonates with subsequent BGL < 2.0 mmol/L, should be treated with 40% buccal dextrose gel 200 mg/kg. Support breast feeding. If BGL ≥ 2.0 mmol/L, breastfeed and/or offer expressed breast milk. For formula fed infants give 10–15 mL/kg in 3 hourly feed volumes. If BGL < 2 mmol/L before the 3rd feed repeat one loop of 40% buccal dextrose gel 200 mg/kg.	Consider oral dextrose gel as an adjunct to a feeding plan in newborn infants at risk of hypoglycemia.	If BGL is 1.5–2.5 mmol/L and baby is ≥35 w, well and feeding, give oral glucose gel 40% and ensure that the baby has an effective feed (feed at least 3 hourly). If BGL 2–2.6 mmol/L, administer a 2nd dose of oral glucose gel 40%. If BGL is <1.5 mmol/L admit the baby to neonatal unit and start IV glucose 10%.	Give 40% dextrose gel 0.5 mL/kg or feed 5 mL/kg and breastfeed. Check glucose 30 min post-feed. To augment caloric intake and before starting IV dextrose, provide enteral supplementation for asymptomatic infants (BGL: 1.9–2.6 mmol/L).	Not discussed
Management of symptomatic NH	Prompt intervention required. Obtain plasma sample for a laboratory glucose determination just before giving an IV "minibolus" of glucose (200 mg of glucose/kg, 2 mL/kg dextrose 10% in water IV) and/or starting a continuous infusion of glucose ($D_{10}W$ at 80–100 mL/kg/day).	If BGL < 1.0 mmol/L and/or clinical signs of NH, obtain IV access, give IV 10% glucose 2.5 mL/kg, start IV infusion of 10% glucose at 60 mL/kg/d. Do not stop breast feeding unless baby too sick to feed or contraindication to enteral feeding. In formula-fed infants, continue feeds if no contraindication. Recheck BGL after 30 min.	If clinical signs or very low BGL, IV dextrose (IV bolus of 2.5 mL/kg 10% glucose) as soon as possible, followed by constant rate glucose infusion.	Not discussed	Administer IV dextrose if not responded to enteral supplementation. If neurological signs, treat immediately with an IV infusion of glucose. Response to IV glucose rechecked after 30 min. If failure to respond, stepwise increase in glucose supply, with a review of levels 30 min after each increment.	IV dextrose infusion. Initial dose: 200 mg/kg, followed by infusion of 10% dextrose at a maintenance rate for age.

Table 2. *Cont.*

	AAP	BAPM	EFCNI	AUS	CPS	PES
Alternative treatments	Not discussed	If unable to obtain immediate IV access, give 40% dextrose gel 200 mg/kg massaged into the buccal mucosa while IV access is obtained or IM glucagon (200 mg/kg).	Not discussed	If BGL not normal after buccal glucose gel 40% or IV glucose, consider: Glucagon (in hyperinsulinemic conditions refractory to IV glucose infusion), hydrocortisone, diazoxide, hydrochlorothiazide, octreotide.	When infusions fail to maintain BG at appropriate levels or an especially high rate (>10 mg/kg/min) of infusion is required, consider further investigation/specialist referral, and/or pharmacological intervention (Glucagon, hydrocortisone, diazoxide, octreotide)	Medications for hyperinsulinism, and cortisol or growth hormone deficiency. Consider surgery for hyperinsulinemic children unable to maintain safe BGL through medical therapy. Nutritional therapy for disorders of glycogen metabolism or hereditary fructose intolerance. Some milder disorders may be treated by avoidance of prolonged fasting.
Target Glucose concentration-Discharge plan	Target PG $\geq$ 45 mg/dL prior to routine feeds. Ensure maintenance of normal PG concentrations on a routine diet for a reasonably extended period (through at least three feed–fast periods) before discharge.	BGL $\geq$ 2.0 mmol/L. Recommended operational threshold: 3.0 mmol/L in neonates with suspected hyperinsulinism < 48 h after birth. Ensure maintenance of BGL > 2.0 mmol/L on $\geq$2 consecutive occasions as well as effective feeding before discharging babies at risk.	Not discussed	Discharge if baby < 48 h of age and pre-prandial BGL > 2.6 mmol/L for three feed–fast cycles or if known hypoglycemic condition and baby $\geq$ 48 h of age and pre-prandial BGL is >4 mmol/L for three feed–fast cycles. A 6 h fast test performed (if indicated) and baby able to maintain BGL.	Target BGL > 2.6 mmol/L for babies younger than 72 h of age and BGL > 3.3 mmol/L for older ones.	Target PG > 70 mg/dL (3.9 mmol/L) for neonates with a suspected congenital hypoglycemic disorder and older infants and children with a hypoglycemic disorder. Target PG > 50 mg/dL (2.8 mmol/L) for high-risk neonates without suspected congenital hypoglycemic disorder aged <48 h and PG > 60 mg/dL (3.3 mmol/L) for those aged >48 h.

NH: neonatal hypoglycemia; PG: plasma glucose; BGL: blood glucose levels; RR: respiratory rate; HR: heart rate; RF: risk factors; T: temperature; NICU: neonatal intensive care unit; IV: intravenous; IM: intramuscular; BG: blood glucose.

3. Definition of Neonatal Hypoglycemia

Many healthy infants experience transient hypoglycemia as part of their normal adaptation to extrauterine life, resulting from the discontinuation of nutrients due to the separation from the placental circulation [5]. This leads to a transient reduction in BGL beginning at 1 to 2 h after birth, known as "physiologic" hypoglycemia (as low as 30 mg/dL (1.6 mmol/L) according to the AAP and BAPM or 20–25 mg/dL (1.1–1.4 mmol/L) according to EFCNI and AUS). The lowest point is usually reached in the first 2 to 4 h of life; at 4 to 6 h, the BGL usually stabilize at 2.5–4.4 mmol/L (45–79 mg/dL) [17]. Glucose is the major oxidative fuel of the brain; however, this transient, asymptomatic form of hypoglycemia can be relatively easily compensated through the production of alternative sources of energy, such as ketone bodies released from fat. After the first 2 postnatal hours, the glucose concentration begins to rise, mainly due to endogenous production (glycogenolysis and gluconeogenesis) rather than feeding. This is the result of a mild and transient form of hyperinsulinism where the mean threshold of BGL for the suppression of insulin secretion is lower in newborn babies (55–65 mg/dL (3.0–3.6 mmol/L)) than in older infants and children (80–85 mg/dL (4.4–4.7 mmol/L)) [18]. The mechanism responsible for the glucose-stimulated insulin secretion matures with age, resulting in an increase in the mean threshold of BGL, which, by 72 h of age, is similar to those in older infants and children [18].

It is common for healthy, breast-fed newborns to present low BGL (<36 mg/dL (2 mmol/L)) during the first 24 h of life [19] without abnormal clinical signs or symptoms. A randomized controlled trial, called "The Sugar Babies Study", which enrolled 514 infants of 35–42 gestational weeks, younger than 48 h old, identified to be at risk for NH, found that 51% of babies became hypoglycemic (BGL < 47 mg/dL (2.6 mmol/L)) and 19% had severe hypoglycemia (BGL < 36 mg/dL (2.0 mmol/L)). The majority of the hypoglycemic ones, i.e., 79%, showed no clinical signs [3]. Given these facts, defining a clinical diagnosis of NH is crucial to provide guidance for when and whether therapy should be initiated.

If any infant shows clinical manifestations compatible with significantly low BGL, such as apnea, jitteriness and seizures, the plasma glucose (PG) or BG concentration should be measured immediately. The AAP and PES support measuring PG levels to define hypoglycemia, while the BAPM, EFCNI, AUS and CPS recommend whole BGL measurement. PG values tend to be higher compared to the whole blood glucose levels by approximately 10–18% (AAP), 10–15% (BAPM, EFCNI), 15% (PES), 10% (CPS), because the concentration of water in the plasma is higher than in the whole blood [18].

However, the definition of NH lacks uniformity among the reviewed guidelines. First, although all societies divide newborns into two groups depending on their postnatal age, to make a distinction between transient and persistent NH, the AUS, BAPM and PES use a cutoff of 48 h, while CPS and EFCNI draw the line at 72 h of age. The PES guideline are based not only on the neonate's age but also on the presence or absence of a known or suspected hypoglycemic congenital disorder, as they mostly address the matter of evaluation and management of persistent NH. Furthermore, the CPS recommends a different cutoff of glucose levels in transient (within the first 72 h of life) than in persistent NH (beyond the first 72 h of life), as the former is defined by BGL lower than 2.6 mmol/L (47 mg/dL) (also endorsed by AUS and AAP), while the latter by BGL lower than 3.3 mmol/L (59 mg/dL). The definition of persistent NH given by the EFCNI is consistent, i.e., NH lasting beyond 72 h of postnatal life. In contrast, the BAPM guidelines define transient NH (during the first 48 h of life) by BGL between 1.0 and 1.9 mmol/L (18–34 mg/dL) documented on one or two occasions, whereas persistent NH (beyond the first 48 h of life) is defined by BGL lower than 2.0 mmol/L (36 mg/dL) on more than two occasions. The AUS and PES also propose the cut-off point of 48 h to distinguish transitional from persistent hypoglycemia and the AUS describes recurrent NH as BGL below 2.6 mmol/L (47 mg/dL) on more than three occasions in a row.

The definition of severe NH is also controversial. More specifically, the BAPM mentions that NH should be characterized as severe when BGL are <1.0 mmol/L (18 mg/dL), while the AUS suggests a definition of BGL < 1.5 mmol/L (27 mg/dL), BGL not recordable or symptomatic hypoglycemia.

This distinction has implications on management as transient NH in the absence of associated clinical manifestations does not require further investigation [20], while severe and persistent NH should prompt urgent medical attention and additional investigations because it may be the first sign of a severe metabolic disorder, like hyperinsulinemic hypoglycemia or hypopituitarism [21].

On the other hand, the term "clinical hypoglycemia" is used by the PES and AUS guidelines to describe the concentration of PG that is low enough to cause brain injury [22].

4. Screening for Neonatal Hypoglycemia

There is no consensus regarding the exact timing when screening should be performed (AAP). Data regarding both the optimal timing and time intervals for screening blood glucose are limited and it remains controversial whether it is necessary to screen the at-risk newborns who do not present any signs or symptoms of NH during the time that BGL reach their normal lowest point (approximately within 1–2 h after delivery) [23]. Furthermore, the evidence supporting routine screening for NH of asymptomatic infants who have no risk factors for hypoglycemia, after a non-complicated pregnancy and delivery, is insufficient.

Five of the reviewed guidelines (AAP, BAPM, EFCNI, AUS, CPS) provide guidance for the screening of NH. They all agree that screening for NH should be performed only for infants with suspected or well-established risk factors for developing hypoglycemia; any infant with abnormal feeding behavior, absence of feeding cues or any other clinical manifestations should be promptly screened for NH at any time; in fact, screening is recommended within minutes, not hours, of the appearance of symptoms and with a duration and frequency of BGL testing that depend on individualized risk factors.

With regard to the initial screening, BAPM, EFCNI and AUS support that the optimal time for screening of asymptomatic, at-risk neonates is just before the second feed (practically no longer than 2–4 h after delivery) provided that the newborn is offered feeding within the first hour after birth. On the contrary, according to AAP and CPS, the recommended time for screening high-risk infants is 30 min after the first feed (practically up to 2 h of age) followed by intervention with feeding or IV glucose depending on the glucose values. The AAP and CPS agree with the BAPM and AUS on the timing of the initial feed, which should be offered to the neonate within the first hour after delivery. Regarding the subsequent BGL measurements, after the initial screening of asymptomatic at-risk infants, all five medical societies agree that measurements should be performed prior to feedings. Breast milk or formula feedings should be offered to newborns every 2–3 h or more frequently.

Furthermore, the AUS and BAPM guidelines suggest a second BGL screening before the third feed and no later than six hours (AUS) or eight hours (BAPM) of age. However, the subsequent steps differ. More specifically, according to the AUS, if BGL is within the normal range ($\geq$2.6 mmol/L, >47 mg/dL), screening should continue to be performed before every second feed (every three to six hours depending on feeding frequency) for 24 h. On the contrary, if the second BGL measurement is above 2.0 mmol/L, the BAPM proposes no further glucose measurements, unless signs or symptoms indicative of hypoglycemia are present, and only recommends observation for 24 h, providing continuous support of breastfeeding. According to the CPS, testing should also be performed one or two times during the second day of life, to ensure that the BGL remain above 2.6 mmol/L (47 mg/dL), whereas the AAP suggests repeated testing prior to feedings after the first 24 h of age only if PG values remain lower than 45 mg/dL (2.5 mmol/L).

Additionally, the AAP and the CPS agree upon continuing measurements through multiple feed–fast cycles depending on the risk factors of each newborn. On the one hand, small-for-gestational-age (SGA) and late-preterm neonates should be screened for at least the first 24 h before each feeding (every 2–3 h); in addition, if the BGL remain above 2.6 mmol/L (47 mg/dL), screening should be discontinued [24]. On the other hand, large-for-gestational-age neonates and those of diabetic mothers should be screened only for the first 12 h after birth, with the same cut-off glucose value used for discontinuing measurements. This difference in the duration of BGL screening is based on studies showing that IDM and LGA infants are more likely to become hypoglycemic by 12 h after the birth, in contrast to preterm and SGA infants, who usually develop asymptomatic NH within 24 h [24–26].

5. Diagnosis of Neonatal Hypoglycemia

Diagnosing NH using a single glucose value is neither feasible nor simple [19]. Thus, monitoring, managing and preventing NH remain highly pressing issues [27]. According to the AUS, CPS and AAP, the generally adopted PG concentration cut-off for otherwise healthy infants is 47 mg/dL (2.6 mmol/L). More specifically, the CPS guideline refers to the existence of four approaches to the diagnosis of NH based on the following aspects: 1. the neonate's clinical condition; 2. epidemiological data from studies on exclusively breastfed, appropriate-for-gestational-age (AGA), term infants and their measured BGL [4,21,28]; 3. the presence or absence of normal physiological responses to NH; and 4. the presence or absence of brain injury and long-term sequelae.

However, as stated by AAP, there is no robust scientific justification for the generally adopted cut-off of blood glucose for NH in all infants (47 mg/dL, 2.6 mmol/L) [23,28] and the normal range of blood glucose concentration in neonates depends on various factors, such as their birthweight, gestational age, clinical manifestations, energy sources and metabolic demands. The reasons that make it difficult to form and adopt a substantial, evidence-based definition for NH and an accurate value for BG that requires intervention in all neonates are the frequent co-existence of other severe medical conditions and the lack of evidence on the levels of BG and the duration of NH that can cause brain injury and long-term neurological sequelae, alone or in concert with comorbidities [4,22].

This is why the approach of the "operational threshold" has been introduced by a panel of experts that convened in 2000 [4] and has been endorsed by all six medical societies to guide interventions intended to restore BGL. An operational threshold constitutes the concentration of BGL (either plasma or whole blood) that should raise awareness of physicians to consider intervention based on evidence available in the current literature, distinguishing between the BG value that requires action and the target BGL that interventions aim for [4]. This "operational threshold" approach has been widely adopted for all neonates at risk of impaired metabolic adaptation and adverse outcome, but the threshold values for whole BG or PG for diagnosis of NH and consequent intervention remain a matter of keen debate.

Thus, according to BAPM, the most important threshold concentrations at which clinicians should consider intervention include: 1. a BG value < 1.0 mmol/L (<18 mg/dL) at any time, 2. a single value < 2.5 mmol/L (45 mg/dL) in a neonate with abnormal clinical signs, and 3. a value < 2.0 mmol/L (36 mg/dL) that remains that low in a subsequent measurement, in case of a newborn with one risk factor for impaired metabolic adaptation but not presenting any abnormal clinical signs and/or symptoms. These thresholds are higher when it comes to symptomatic newborn infants with recurrent or persistent hyperinsulinemic hypoglycemia (HH). In such cases, therapeutic levels of 3.0 mmol/L (54 mg/dL) or more are suggested [12]. According to AUS, any neonate with BGL < 1.5 mmol/L or unrecordable measurement, as well as any symptomatic neonate, requires urgent management and further investigation, while the value used as an operational threshold is BGL below 2.6 mmol/L (47 mg/dL) in all at risk neonates. The PES recommends PG levels to be kept >2.8 mmol/L (50 mg/dL) during the first 48 h of postnatal life and >3.3 mmol/L (60 mg/dL) after 48 h for high-risk neonates without a suspected congenital hypoglycemic disorder. The same operational threshold for blood glucose but in a different time window (after 72 h of life) is recommended by the CPS guidelines, while for the first 72 h postpartum, the CPS suggests the threshold glucose value of 2.0 mmol/L, for which further management is required. The PES recommend that the operational threshold for neonates with a suspected congenital or confirmed hypoglycemic disorder is higher, as in such cases the PG must be maintained >70 mg/dL (3.9 mmol/L), in contrast with 3.0 mmol/L suggested by the BAPM and 3.3 mmol/L by the AUS. Moreover, PES defines the considered-to-be-normal PG values for neonates as 55–65 mg/dL in the first 48 h of age and 70–100 mg/dL for older ones. The AAP recommends operational thresholds for PG concentration in high-risk newborns that differ depending on the hours of age: 25–40 mg/dL (1.4–2.2 mmol/L), 35–45 mg/dL (1.9–2.5 mmol/L) and 45 mg/dL (2.5 mmol/L), from birth to 4 h of life, from 4–24 h of life and after 24 h of life, respectively. The AAP also recommends intervention for all neonates with clinical signs and a PG concentration less than 40 mg/dL. Finally, the EFCNI, adopts the operational threshold approach on guiding interventions and clinical decisions based on glucose values approved by professionals in all maternity and neonatal units; however, they underline the profound controversy among recommendations of different organizations, due to the lack of evidence-based data on cerebral damage provoked by NH [29]. Thus, the EFCNI does not specifically define NH, only stating that BGL as low as 1.0 mmol/L (18 mg/dL) are associated with acute neurological impairment [9,23].

6. Diagnostic Methods of Neonatal Hypoglycemia

The accurate measurement of BGL is crucial for the diagnosis and treatment of NH. Therefore, the optimal methods of BGL assessment are discussed in all guidelines reviewed. Blood glucose levels are usually measured using chemical strips or bedside handheld glucose meters (non-enzymatic methods) and most of the time they are not validated using laboratory diagnostic tests [15,30].

However, the accuracy of bedside reagent test-strip glucose analyzers is limited, especially in the low range of BG concentrations. This low range is defined as 10–15 mg/dL (0.6–0.8 mmol/L) by the PES, and as 0–36 mg/dL (0–2.0 mmol/L) by the BAPM and EFCNI, whereas no specific values are provided by the other societies. It is also crucial to keep in mind that the neonatal packed cell volume (PCV) could be a cause of inaccuracy in handheld glucometers due to the fact that they do not auto-correct for this variable. Samples with high PCV can generate falsely low glucose values and vice versa [12]. Moreover, even though only few devices that measure true whole BG values by rupturing red blood cells are available, most handheld test-strip glucometers report results that demonstrate a reasonable correlation with PG concentrations and that are considered to be "PG equivalents". Whole BG and PG levels may vary up to 10 to 20 mg/dL, but the gap becomes wider at low glucose concentrations.

These are the reasons why these point of care methods are not reliable enough to be used as the sole method for NH screening [30,31], as highlighted by all six guidelines. More specifically, the AAP, PES, CPS and AUS guidelines state that the initial screening could be performed using "rapid" bedside tests (including handheld reflectance colorimeter and electrode methods validated for neonatal samples), to prevent any delay for the rapid diagnosis and initiation of treatment, provided that the clinician is aware of their limited accuracy. Capillary samples obtained from a warmed heel can be used for screening, as agreed by all these guidelines.

However, due to the limitations of these handheld glucometer devices, before establishing a diagnosis of NH, glucose concentration (plasma or whole blood) must be confirmed using laboratory enzymatic methods (glucose oxidase, hexokinase and dehydrogenase methods). According to AAP, although not rapidly available, laboratory testing is the most accurate method for BGL measuring. The AUS specifies that, if the initial screening of BGL is <2.6 mmol/L (47 mg/dL) in neonates with clinical manifestations compatible with hypoglycemia or with risk factors for NH, glucose values should be validated using point-of-care diagnostic tests (such as enzymatic handheld glucometers with glucose oxidase or glucose dehydrogenase methodology, if available), blood gas analyzers or laboratory enzymatic methods (in fluoride oxalate tube, if feasible to be performed immediately). The same diagnostic methods are recommended by the AUS, in case of initial BGL < 2.0 mmol/L (36 mg/dL), in all newborn infants. As delineated by the AUS, AAP and CPS guidelines, treatment should not be delayed while waiting for the results to be confirmed using a laboratory test, especially for severe, persistent or recurrent NH [4]. Additionally, the CPS guideline mentions another diagnostic method for NH, called CGMs (continuous glucose monitors), which, however, have numerous limitations that question their accuracy; the development of other more promising and more accurate point-of-care devices for bedside glucose measurement may improve the screening methods for NH. On the contrary, the BAPM and EFCNI state that blood gas analyzers are quick, widely available and accurate for measuring BG values. Furthermore, they calculate glucose result as "PG equivalent" concentration, which in most cases is similar to the result obtained from a laboratory enzymatic diagnostic method. Thus, blood gas biosensors are considered to be the gold standard in the screening of NH, as they support real-time clinical decision making and they could be set up to provide a 'glucose only' reading on a tiny neonatal blood sample [32]. If handheld glucometers are used (necessarily compliant with the specific ISO15197:2013 standard), it is highly important for clinicians to remember their limitations in accuracy at low BGL and to confirm their results with more accurate techniques to ensure that hypoglycemic infants are assigned to the optimal care pathway. As stated by the BAPM, a laboratory confirmation may not be practical, not only because of the delay in obtaining results but also due to inconsistency of the results, caused by variability in the inhibition of glycolysis in fluoride oxalate tubes. Lastly, a new technology—currently under development—based on transdermal, minimally invasive, constant and accurate blood sugar measurements provided by biosensors is discussed in the BAPM guidelines as a very promising useful tool for future research [33].

7. Prevention

There is general agreement on the basic principles of NH prevention among the BAPM, EFCNI, AUS and CPS guidelines. These include the following: 1. the antenatal or immediate postnatal identification of all at-risk infants; 2. the avoidance of cold stress and hypothermia—ideally by providing skin to skin contact with the mother; 3. the early and timely energy provision and feeding support; 4. the regular BGL monitoring at predetermined times with accurate devices that provide results with no delay; 5. the constant observation of both the feeding behavior and the overall clinical condition of the neonate; and 6. a thorough discussion with the parents regarding the neonate's feeding and well-being. The BAPM, EFCNI and AUS guidelines describe these principals in detail. On the other hand, the AAP does not mention any measures for the prevention of NH, the CPS focuses on the neonate's feeding standards to prevent NH, and the PES only refers to disorders with persistent NH, such as hyperinsulinism, in which the main goal of prevention is trying to avoid recurrent episodes of hypoglycemia that may increase the risk of subsequent, possibly unrecognized hypoglycemic episodes.

Clinicians should keep in mind that early recognition is vital to avoid serious health disorders and improve outcomes. First, the risk factors for NH must be identified at birth to provide meticulous care and extra support to the newborns. More specifically, the AUS highlights that preterm infants of ≤35 gestational weeks should be admitted to neonatal units and receive special care by managing other possible co-existing clinical conditions, ensuring thermal care and providing early and frequent feeds, assisted with gavage if needed or indicated for neonates not nippling well (AAP, AUS, BAPM).

Additionally, a thorough and regular assessment of the neonate's clinical condition when awake is important. The general appearance, muscle tone, body measurements, body malformations or deformations (indicative of a syndrome potentially responsible for NH), skin color, body temperature (normal range within 36.5–37.5 °C measured via the axilla), level of consciousness, response to external stimulations, respiratory and heart rate and all feeding cues should be evaluated [10]. Abnormal feeding behaviors that should raise awareness and call for action include not waking for meals, not latching at the breast, not sucking effectively and appearing unsettled. The BAPM and AUS guidelines point out that when signs or symptoms suggestive of NH make their appearance, BGL should be immediately measured and a pediatrician or a neonatal nurse practitioner should be called for assistance and further guidance.

Moreover, the BAPM, EFCNI and AUS thoroughly describe all the steps that should be followed to prevent hypothermia of the at-risk neonate, including the use of a hat, the avoidance of cold draughts, the warmth of the ambient temperature and the immediate skin-to-skin contact with the mother, while the CPS suggests that the first bath should be delayed for at-risk infants as it has been found to decrease the incidence of NH [34].

The crucial role of the parents in the monitoring and management of infants at risk for impaired metabolic adaptation is highlighted by three of the reviewed guidelines (BAPM, CPS and EFCNI). They point out that parents should participate actively in the care pathway of at-risk neonates, being aware not only of the reasons behind their newborns' requirement of extra care and why they undergo regular blood testing for measuring BGL, but also of all the signs and symptoms that could indicate hypoglycemia. Thus, parents can learn about the importance of early energy provision and help physicians with BG monitoring. If risk factors for NH are known before delivery, health care providers should communicate with the parents to inform them antenatally. The BAPM suggests that this information should be given to parents in both verbal and written form, while the EFCNI suggests giving this information only verbally.

The BAPM, EFCNI, AUS and CPS note that breast milk is the optimal source of energy for all neonates during their postpartum metabolic adaptation. The early initiation of feeds plays a significant role in preventing NH and it should be ensured that the neonate is offered the breast within the first 60 min (BAPM) or 30–60 min (AUS) of life [10,35]. Efficient support should be provided to all mothers to make them feel capable of initiating and establishing effective breastfeeding and to enable them to recognize both early feeding cues and signs of effective attachment. Feeding effectiveness should be assessed at each feed and the breastfeeding should be offered at least 8–10 times in 24 h, according to feeding cues. As stated by the BAPM, there should not exist a gap of more than three hours between the meals until BGL exceeds 2 mmol/L (36 mg/dL) on two or more consecutive measurements [12]. The main goal is to cover the neonate's energy demands as much as possible using breast milk or expressed colostrum/breast milk.

In formula-fed infants, the timing of initial feed and time intervals between feedings are practically the same. The AUS guideline supports that complementary feeds are not required in the first 24 h of life, unless one BGL measurement is <2 mmol/L (36 mg/dL) or two or more BGL values are <2.6 mmol/L (47 mg/dL), whereas it mentions that if formula feeding is chosen, meals should be up to 60–75 mL/kg/day for at-risk newborns. In cases where complementary feeds are required, a minimum of 7.5 mL/kg/feed should be provided [10]. The CPS guidelines differ in that they suggest supplementing feeds with breast milk or a breast milk substitute; the total volume of both oral and IV intake should not exceed 100 mL/kg/day so as to avoid fluid overload and serum electrolytes disorders. This medical society also highlights the importance of continuing to feed high-risk infants regularly, while continuing to measure BGL prior to meals, as well as the use of a pump to achieve slow feeding (breast milk or formula) rather than bolus feeding.

8. Management of Asymptomatic Neonatal Hypoglycemia

The goals of managing NH are as follows: first, to identify at risk newborns and newborns with serious underlying hypoglycemic disorders [36]; second, to correct BGL; and third, to avoid unnecessary treatment of normal transitional NH, which will likely resolve without intervention [37]. It is crucial to keep in mind that the treatment of hypoglycemia is a stepwise process depending on the presence or absence of symptoms and signs and on the infant's response at each step. All of the reviewed guidelines highlight the importance of recognizing and treating asymptomatic NH early and agree on the main principles of management, which are as follows: 1. the antenatal or immediate postpartum identification of risk factors, 2. the provision of thermal care, 3. the early energy provision and feeding support, 4. the regular monitoring of BGL and infusion of IV dextrose when necessary, and 5. to try not to interrupt the mother–infant relationship and breastfeeding when possible.

For asymptomatic newborns at risk, the AAP suggests a treatment plan that is divided into two time periods, up to 4 h of age and between 4 and 24 h of age. An initial feed should be offered to all neonates within the first hour of age and an initial screen of BGL should be performed 30 min after the first feed. If the PG is <25 mg/dL (1.3 mmol/L), another feeding-checking PG in a one hour-cycle is recommended, and if PG remains <25 mg/dL, IV glucose administration is indicated (glucose dose 200 mg/kg, 2 mL/kg dextrose 10% D/W). If the PG is between 25 and 40 mg/dL (1.3–2.2 mmol/L), another attempt to feed may be made before progressing with glucose administration [38]. For newborns aged 4 to 24 h, feeding every 2–3 h (after the initial feed) and PG measurements prior to each feed are recommended. If PG is <35 mg/dL (1.9 mmol/L) in one sample, it is suggested to refeed and recheck PG concentration within 1 h. If PG remains <3 5 mg/dL, intravenous glucose should be administered (same dose as before). However, if PG is between 35 and 45 mg/dL (1.9–2.5 mmol/L), active support of feeding should continue before the initiation of treatment with IV dextrose solution.

According to the BAPM and AUS guidelines, at-risk neonates should be placed in two care pathways based on their first pre-feed BGL. For the BAPM, the first cut-off point is BGL between 1.0 and 1.9 mmol/L (18–34 mg/dL) in infants with no abnormal clinical signs, while the second cut-off point is either BGL < 1.0 mmol/L (18 mg/dL) in neonates without clinical manifestations or higher BGL but with neonates showing symptoms consistent with NH. For the AUS, the cut-off points are as follows: 1. BGL between 1.5 and 2.5 mmol/L (27–45 mg/dL) in asymptomatic neonates; and 2. BGL below 1.5 mmol/L (27 mg/dL) or unrecordable values or symptomatic neonates within the first 48 h of life.

The BAPM suggests that when BGL are between 1.0 and 1.9 mmol/L (18–34 mg/dL) and no clinical manifestations are present, the administration of 40% oral dextrose gel (dose of 200 mg/kg) should be considered as part of the feeding plan, alongside breastfeeding or formula feeding, if the mother chooses so. The AUS recommendations for at-risk asymptomatic infants with BGL 1.5–2.5 mmol/L (27–45 mg/dL) and the CPS recommendations for at-risk infants with BGL < 2.6 mmmol/L (47 mg/dL) agree with those of the BAPM, as a dose of 40% dextrose gel is suggested to be given buccally (dose of 0.5 mL/kg equivalent to 200 mg/kg) in conjunction with oral feedings. The EFCNI also aligns with the aforementioned guidelines on this matter, as it is generally stated that oral dextrose gel may be considered as an adjunct to a feeding plan in high-risk newborns. This oral 40% dextrose gel of 0.5 mL/kg provides a dose of 200 mg/kg glucose, which is equivalent to the intravenous bolus glucose dose of 2 mL/kg of the 10% DW solution. Its administration is indicated only in late preterm and term infants (CPS) or neonates > 35 weeks of gestational age (BAPM, AUS) during the first 48 h after delivery, with a maximum of six doses during this period of time (AUS, BAPM). The "Sugar Babies" study, which is described in the CPS and BAPM guidelines, assessed the effectiveness of dextrose oral gel treatment over feeding alone in hypoglycemic neonates and showed that therapy with dextrose gel leads to significant lower treatment failure rates compared to placebo. The buccal gel has also been found to reduce the number of NICU admissions due to NH, alongside the need for supplementation with formula at 2 weeks of age [39]. In fact, if glucose gel administration is followed by immediate breastfeeding, the quality of subsequent breast feeds is improved [40]. However, although it decreases the need for IV glucose administration, it cannot achieve the complete avoidance of IV therapy [39].

Furthermore, according to the BAPM, BG should be measured again prior to the third feed and no longer than 8 h of age, and if BGL fail to rise above 2 mmol/L (36 mg/dL), another circle of oral dextrose gel and feeding should be repeated. A re-check of BGL is also recommended by the AUS (30 min after the first dose of oral dextrose gel) and a subsequent dose of dextrose gel is considered safe to be administered if the BGL remain between 2.0 and 2.5 mmol/L (36–45 mg/dL). Similarly, according to CPS, BGL should be re-measured 30 min post-feed and if they remain between 1.9 and 2.6 mmol/L (34–47 mg/dL), another loop of oral dextrose gel 40% (same dosage) followed by enteral supplementation (breastfeeding or formula feeding) and a glucose measurement again 30 min after feeding is recommended. On the contrary, if BGL are <1.9 mmol/L (34 mg/dL) (CPS), 1.0 mmol/L (18 mg/dL) (BAPM) or 1.5 mmol/L (AUS), the initiation of IV glucose infusion at hourly requirements (10% DW) is strongly advised without repeating the loop of oral dextrose gel–breastfeeding/formula feeding/EBM.

In addition, if more than two measurements between 1.0 and 1.9 mmol/L have been documented or if two consecutive doses of glucose gel 40% have been given, the neonatal team should be informed to investigate possible causes of NH and to exclude other disorders that mimic hypoglycemia, like sepsis. Admission to the Neonatal Intensive Care Unit (NICU) is required (BAPM, AUS) in such cases. An increase in the feeding frequency and the insertion of a nasogastric tube should also be considered and the IV glucose administration (10% DW) at this point is suggested, too. It is important to remember that buccal dextrose gel can be used as first-line treatment for hypoglycemia, allowing the infant–mother relationship not to be interrupted, avoiding NICU hospitalization and improving the chances of effective breastfeeding after discharge [39].

Additionally, as stated by the BAPM, if BGL are >2.0 mmol/L, breastfeeding or formula feeding and/or EBM should continue to be offered, glucose should be measured again prior to the next feed, and if BGL remain >2.0 mmol/L (after two consecutive pre-feed BG measurements) and no clinical manifestations are present, it is advised that BG measurements are discontinued. According to the AUS, the conditions under which cessation of BGL monitoring is indicated are as follows: (a) BGL $\geq$ 2.6 mmol/L or $\geq$3.3 mmol/L for 24 h, within or beyond the first 48 h of life, respectively, (b) neonate feeding effectively, (c) asymptomatic neonate for whom IV glucose had not been required. For neonates who were treated with IV dextrose but are now feeding well and have not received IV glucose during the past 12 h, monitoring should be ceased when BGL exceed 3 mmol/L for two successive measurements. CPS suggest ceasing pre-feed glucose monitoring when two consecutive BG samples are above 2.6 mmol/L and the neonate fully tolerates enteral feeds.

9. Management of Symptomatic Neonatal Hypoglycemia

The appearance of hypoglycemic clinical signs and symptoms constitutes a red flag for the urgent initiation of therapy because severe, prolonged, symptomatic hypoglycemia may result in neuronal injury [38,41]. First, a laboratory confirmation of the low BGL must always be performed before starting IV treatment, according to the AAP, BAPM and AUS, because it is essential for both the identification and the optimal management of hypoglycemia. However, therapy should not be delayed while waiting for laboratory results. Blood samples during the hypoglycemic period should be collected to perform further diagnostic evaluation [42].

The recommendations of AAP in symptomatic infants with BGL < 40 mg/dL (2.2 mmol/L) involve immediate IV glucose treatment either as an IV bolus glucose dose of 200 mg/kg (2 mL/kg 10% DW) or as an IV glucose infusion of 80–100 mL/kg 10% DW per day to maintain PG concentrations between 40 and 50 mg/dL (2.2–2.7 mmol/L). The CPS guideline agrees with this approach of immediately treating symptomatic infants or infants who cannot be orally fed, with an IV infusion of 10% DW or a bolus IV glucose administration (dose of 2 mL/kg over 15 min) when BGL are lower than 1.8 mmol/L. The administration of a bolus dose at the start of a glucose infusion therapy is believed to stabilize BGL more rapidly. The PES instructions also align with this treatment for any episode of severe symptomatic hypoglycemia with IV dextrose infusion at an initial dose of 200 mg/kg, followed by infusion of 10% DW at a maintenance rate. A response to the intravenous administration of glucose is expected in the next 30 min and a confirmation should be performed in a timely manner [43].

The recommendations of EFCNI and BAPM on symptomatic hypoglycemia or newborns presenting with very low glucose levels (<1.0 mmol/L, 18 mg/dL) are consistent, as they suggest that in such cases infants should be treated with IV glucose as an initial bolus of 2.5 mL/kg 10%DW (instead of 2 mL/kg 10%DW) as soon as possible, followed by a glucose infusion administration of 60 mL/kg 10% DW per day (instead of 80–100 mL/kg/day). The recommended of the AUS for initial IV bolus glucose dose for symptomatic newborns or BGL below 1.5 mmol/L (27 mg/dL) is 1–2 mL/kg 10% DW, followed by the re-measurement of BGL in the next 30 min and repeated by another bolus glucose dose of 1 mL/kg IV while monitoring for rebound hypoglycemia. The IV glucose infusion rate should commence at 60 mL/kg/day 10% DW. The AUS also gives instructions for treating newborns with BGL between 1.5 and 2.5 mmol/L who are not feeding well (symptomatic newborns). In such cases, one dose of 40% oral dextrose gel should be given, a neonatal nurse practitioner or a pediatrician should be informed, a lactation consultant should be notified and BGL should be re-measured within 30 min. If the BGL are between 2.0 and 2.6 mmol/L, a second dose of 40% oral dextrose gel can be administered and breastfeeding or formula feeding and/or EBM should be continued. If the BGL are <2 mmol/L, the neonate must be admitted to the NICU in order to initiate IV treatment.

There is a consensus among the reviewed guidelines that for the management of symptomatic NH, an intravenous access should be obtained (peripheral or central). The AUS points out that in case the required IV glucose infusion concentration is more than 12%, an umbilical venous catheter or central line should be inserted; however, the CPS question previous data that dictated the need for a central vein for glucose solutions with concentration $\geq$ 15% and supports the integrity of peripheral veins with dextrose concentrations up to 20% based on a randomized controlled trial of 121 hypoglycemic newborns, which showed that 20% and 15% glucose solutions can be infused equally safely into peripheral veins in neonates [44]. Nevertheless, in case an IV access is not easy or possible to be established immediately, two alternatives are proposed as urgent interventions: 40% dextrose gel 200 mg/kg equivalent to 0.5 mL/kg- administered orally via buccal massage (BAPM), or intramuscular injection of glucagon 200 microgram/kg (BAPM, AUS, CPS). It is important, however, to keep in mind that if the BGL are <1.0 mmol/L, the buccal dextrose gel should only be used as an interim measure while trying to establish an IV line [45].

The continuation of treatment is based on the regular assessment of the neonatal clinical condition and its BGL monitoring. The PES, AAP and EFCNI guidelines do not discuss in detail the next steps of the neonate's ongoing management, whereas the BAPM, AUS and CPS recommendations agree that if the first intervention is followed by failure to raise BGL, a stepwise increase in glucose supply may be necessary. The AUS recommends that the glucose rate should be daily increased by 20 mL/kg, without exceeding the total daily fluid intake of 100 mL/kg on the first day of life, to prevent fluid overload. The concentration of the IV dextrose solution could also be increased from 10% DW to 12% or higher, keeping in mind the necessity to always measure BGL after any changes to glucose concentration. The same applies to the increase in the glucose delivery rate proposed by BAPM (mentioned as a rise of 2 mg/kg/min) either by increasing the volume or the concentration of IV dextrose solution. At this point, these medical societies agree that if the glucose infusion rate (GIR) is higher than 8 mg/kg/min in the first 24 h after delivery (or, according to BAPM, if BGL is <2.0 mmol/L on more than two measurements during the first 48 h of life), a clinical suspicion of hyperinsulinism should be raised and treatment with glucagon should be commenced. BGL should be measured again in the next 30 min.

According to the BAPM, if the BGL remain <1.0 mmol/L or there are abnormal clinical signs, another cycle of treatment should be repeated with IV bolus 10% DW (2.5 mL/kg), followed by an increase in the glucose infusion delivery rate and re-measurement of BGL 30 min afterwards. If the BGL are between 1.0 and 2.5 mmol/L with no abnormal clinical manifestations, the GIR is suggested to increase by 2 mg/kg/min without another IV bolus dextrose administration, and feedings should continue unless there are contraindications. If the BGL are >2.5 mmol/L, a slow and gradual weaning of IV infusion should start and the enteral feeds should also continue. It is necessary to continue BGL monitoring until the infant is on full enteral feeds and the BGL are >2.5 mmol/L (or 3.0 mmol/L in cases of hyperinsulinism) for several fast–feed cycles during the first 24 h of life.

10. Alternative Treatments

The use of alternative medications for the management of NH in cases where BGL do not become normal after the administration of IV glucose or 40% buccal dextrose gel is addressed by the CPS, PES, BAPM and AUS guidelines. The decision for a long-term therapy for hypoglycemic disorders (either persistent or recurrent) should be made in consultation with an experienced neonatologist, a pediatric endocrinologist or a pediatric metabolic specialist in cases where either glucose infusion rate is very high (>10 mg/kg/min according to CPS or >8 mg/kg/min according to the AUS) or glucose infusions fail to maintain the BGL at acceptable levels (more than two blood sugar measurements of 1.0–1.9 mmol/L during the first 48 h postnatally according to the BAPM; greater than 2.6 mmol/L up to 48 h of age or 3.3 mmol/L after the first 48 h, according to the AUS). Blood samples for further investigations (such as serum cortisol and insulin) should be collected immediately while the newborn remains hypoglycemic before administering any medications because recurrent or persistent NH may be the first sign of an underlying disorder associated with the metabolism of glucose, such as hyperinsulinism, disorders leading to cortisol and growth hormone deficiency and inborn errors of metabolism [42,46]. Regarding these alternatives to glucose administration, the AUS and CPS suggest the utilization of glucagon, hydrocortisone, diazoxide and octreotide, while the AUS also proposes hydrochlorothiazide and the BAPM only mentions glucagon as an alternative when an IV line is difficult to be accessed. On the other hand, PES discourages non-specific treatment with glucocorticoids for NH and recommends the use of glucagon, surgical intervention and nutritional therapies.

Glucagon stimulates gluconeogenesis and glycogenolysis and it can result in raising BGL in term and preterm hypoglycemic infants (AUS, PES, CPS). The CPS guideline states that glucagon may be given via IV bolus or infusion, whereas the AUS, BAPM and PES point out that an intramuscular or subcutaneous injection could be considered—apart from IV administration—if it is not possible or easy to establish an IV access [47]. The IV infusion of glucagon is preferred by the AUS because it prevents an exaggerated stimulation of the pancreas due to a high glucose infusion rate and it does not interfere with the effective establishment of breastfeeding. Additionally, the AUS does not align with the PES regarding the onset of action and duration of glucagon, as the former supports that the BGL rise within one hour upon administration and last, approximately, up to two hours [47], while the latter indicates that the BGL increase within 10–15 min and remain at these levels for at least 1 h. Hypoglycemia non-responsive to glucagon may be provoked by glycogen storage disease [48].

Moreover, hydrocortisone is proposed as an alternative treatment for NH by the AUS and CPS because its mechanism of action includes the stimulation of gluconeogenesis and the reduction in glucose utilization in peripheral tissues. It is remarkable that hydrocortisone has a slower response than glucagon [49]. Hydrocortisone may be preferred when hyponatremia is suspected, the infant is hypotensive, evidence indicative of hypoadrenalism is present or the response to previously administered glucagon is insufficient.

Diazoxide is a potassium channel activator used in cases of persistent NH as long-term management. Its mechanism of action is the inhibition of pancreatic insulin release and can be used in conjunction with hydrochlorothiazide in order to achieve weaning from glucose infusion. Hydrochlorothiazide (proposed as an alternative treatment by the AUS) is a diuretic, which has a mechanism of action similar to the one of diazoxide.

Octreotide is a pharmacological analog to natural somatostatin, usually recommended for known or suspected cases of hyperinsulinemic hypoglycemia, and not indicated for the newborn period.

When medical therapy fails to maintain the BGL in a safe range, surgical intervention is proposed by the PES for neonates with hyperinsulinemic hypoglycemia. The importance of nutritional therapy is emphasized by the PES, especially for disorders of glycogen metabolism or hereditary fructose intolerance.

Although it is not a pharmacological intervention, the AUS describes the increase in fluid volume as an effective alternative measure to manage severe, persistent or recurrent NH. Increasing the volume of IV glucose prior to increasing the concentration of glucose to 12% will result in an immediate change in glucose delivery rate whilst a solution of increased glucose concentration is prepared. In particular, a rise of 20 mL/kg/day in the total volume fluids (which does not exceed the maximum daily fluid intake) leads to an approximate 33% increase in BGL. The maximum tolerated total fluid intake is 100 mL/kg/day for most babies of less than 24 h of age, without being at risk of fluid overload. Serum electrolytes should be monitored within regular intervals in order to avoid hyponatremia and over-hydration.

11. Target Glucose Concentration and Discharge Plan

The reviewed guidelines, based on the physiology of normal neonatal glucose homeostasis, the normal age-related increase in glucose concentrations over the first few days of life, and the various pathophysiological conditions that may result in clinical hypoglycemia recommend steps of treatment in order to initiate therapy in a timely manner and to avoid the complications of NH. This treatment is a long process that depends on BG or PG measurements, the presence or absence of symptoms and/or signs and the infant's clinical response, too. Glucose target values vary among these guidelines, alongside with the discharge criteria of at-risk neonates.

The AAP recommends that the target PG concentration should be >45 mg/dL (2.5 mmol/L) pre-prandially and that neonates should be capable of maintaining normal PG values throughout at least three feed–fast periods of time. The BAPM suggests that the therapeutic goal should be a BGL value > 2.0 mmol/L (36 mg/dL). The AUS states that the BGL target for neonates younger than 48 h of age is >2.6 mmol/L (47 mg/dL) for three feed–fast cycles, while for those older than 48 h with a known hypoglycemic disorder, the target is >4.0 mmol/L (72 mg/dL) for three feed–fast cycles. The CPS supports that the BGL target for newborns younger than 72 h should be >2.6 mmol/L (47 mg/dL) and for newborns older than 72 h > 3.3 mmol/L (60 mg/dL). Finally, the PES states that neonates with a suspected hypoglycemic congenital disorder, as well as older infants and children, should have BGL > 70 mg/dL (3.9 mmol/L) to achieve the therapeutic goal. For high-risk neonates without a congenital hypoglycemic disorder, the target value of PG is >50 mg/dL (2.8 mmol/L) or >60 mg/dL (3.3 mmol/L) for those up to 48 h of age and for those older than 48 h, respectively. The therapeutic target for glucose levels is not discussed by the EFCNI.

With regard to the discharge plan, the BAPM and EFCNI agree that newborns should not be discharged until at least two consecutive pre-prandial glucose measurements are within the normal range and neonates have been feeding effectively over several fast–feed cycles. BAPM clarifies that pre-feed BG measurements should be >2.0 mmol/L for neonates with initial BGL measurements between 1.0 and 1.9 mmol/L and no clinical signs, and >2.5 mmol/L (or 3.0 mmol/L) for neonates with initial BGL below 1.0 mmol/L with/without clinical signs in order to cease monitoring. The AAP states that neonates should maintain normal PG concentrations for at least three feed–fast periods before discharge. The AUS aligns with the recommendations of PES on the management and follow- up of neonates (older than 48 h of age) with a known or suspected cause of persistent or prolonged hypoglycemic disorder or with clinically significant NH (requiring a GIR > 6 mg/kg/min or medication such as diazoxide or hydrochlorothiazide), proposing a safety test of six hours of fasting with regular BG measurements in the interval. This fasting test should be performed after consultation with a pediatric endocrinologist or metabolic specialist and should take place before discharge from nursery to ensure that high-risk neonates are capable of remaining normoglycemic if a feeding is missed, as well as to identify infants who need further investigation and additional management for a persistent hypoglycemic disorder.

12. Conclusions

To summarize, there is an overall agreement among the reviewed guidelines regarding the risk factors associated with NH, the wide variety of non-specific clinical manifestations and the main principles of NH prevention. All medical societies underline that the timely identification of hypoglycemic neonates and immediate initiation of treatment are crucial in preventing permanent brain injury. In addition, the AAP, BAPM, EFCNI, AUS and CPS recommend screening for NH using BG measurement for all symptomatic neonates as well as for all asymptomatic high-risk ones. The diagnosis of NH should be confirmed via laboratory tests; however, a single BG value cannot accurately define NH. Thus, all guidelines endorse the "operational threshold approach" for the management of subsequent interventions.

On the other hand, there is inconsistency concerning the screening algorithms, the definition of NH, the threshold values of glucose for the diagnosis of NH and the treatment protocols of asymptomatic hypoglycemic newborns. Minor discrepancies were also identified regarding the initial intravenous bolus dose of glucose, the following rate of continuous infusion and the alternative therapies of symptomatic neonates as well as the treatment targets. It should be noted that one of the major limitations of this descriptive review, which may partially explain the inconsistency identified across the different medical organizations, is that NH represents a complex condition which may occur due to a variety of causes.

The controversy of the guidelines regarding the management of NH and the lack of universal applicability due to inconsistent definitions and the paucity of a substantial body of evidence is clearly outlined. However, NH remains one of the most common and severe metabolic disturbances in perinatal medicine, with destructive consequences when left untreated. This descriptive review attempts to distill the burgeoning literature and place emphasis on the importance of adopting and implementing consistent international protocols for the definition, diagnosis, operational thresholds, prevention and treatment of NH, with the goal of assisting healthcare providers in best managing hypoglycemic neonates and subsequently minimize the rates of associated neonatal morbidity and mortality. New evidence is constantly being published and the understanding of NH is evolving; further large-scale randomized studies are required to validate and modify the diagnostic and therapeutic approaches suggested by the guidelines.

Author Contributions: Conceptualization, T.D. and I.T.; Methodology, S.G. and M.G.; Validation, A.M. and A.A.; Investigation, S.G.; Resources, M.G.; Data Curation, A.D.; Writing—Original Draft Preparation, M.G.; Writing—Review and Editing, S.G. and T.D.; Visualization, I.T. and A.M.; Supervision, I.T. and A.A.; Project Administration, A.A. and T.D. All authors have read and agreed to the published version of the manuscript.

Funding: This research received no external funding.

Institutional Review Board Statement: Not applicable.

Informed Consent Statement: Not applicable.

Data Availability Statement: Data are publicly available.

Conflicts of Interest: The authors declare no conflict of interest.

References

1. Abramowski, A.; Ward, R.; Hamdan, A.H. *Neonatal Hypoglycemia*; StatPearls: Treasure Island, FL, USA, 2022.
2. Deshpande, S.; Upton, M.; Hawdon, J. *Admissions of Term Newborn Infants for Hypoglycaemia: Their Characteristics and Preventability*; The Neonatal Society: Edinburgh, UK, 2016.
3. Harris, D.L.; Weston, P.J.; Harding, J.E. Incidence of Neonatal Hypoglycemia in Babies Identified as at Risk. *J. Pediatr.* **2012**, *161*, 787–791. [CrossRef] [PubMed]

4. Cornblath, M.; Hawdon, J.M.; Williams, A.F.; Aynsley-Green, A.; Ward-Platt, M.P.; Schwartz, R.; Kalhan, S.C. Controversies Regarding Definition of Neonatal Hypoglycemia: Suggested Operational Thresholds. *Pediatrics* **2000**, *105*, 1141–1145. [CrossRef] [PubMed]
5. Hawdon, J. Postnatal metabolic adaptation and neonatal hypoglycaemia. *Paediatr. Child Health* **2016**, *26*, 135–139. [CrossRef]
6. Shah, R.; Harding, J.; Brown, J.; McKinlay, C. Faculty Opinions recommendation of Neonatal Glycaemia and Neurodevelopmental Outcomes: A Systematic Review and Meta-Analysis. *Neonatology* **2019**, *115*, 116–126. [CrossRef] [PubMed]
7. Burns, C.M.; Rutherford, M.A.; Boardman, J.P.; Cowan, F.M. Patterns of Cerebral Injury and Neurodevelopmental Outcomes After Symptomatic Neonatal Hypoglycemia. *Pediatrics* **2008**, *122*, 65–74. [CrossRef] [PubMed]
8. Vannucci, R.C.; Vannucci, S.J. Hypoglycemic brain injury. *Semin. Neonatol.* **2001**, *6*, 147–155. [CrossRef] [PubMed]
9. Boluyt, N.; van Kempen, A.; Offringa, M. Neurodevelopment After Neonatal Hypoglycemia: A Systematic Review and Design of an Optimal Future Study. *Pediatrics* **2006**, *117*, 2231–2243. [CrossRef]
10. Hawdon, J.M.; Beer, J.; Sharp, D.; Upton, M. Neonatal hypoglycaemia: Learning from claims. *Arch. Dis. Child. Fetal Neonatal Ed.* **2017**, *102*, F110–F115. [CrossRef]
11. Adamkin, D.H. Committee on Fetus and Newborn Postnatal Glucose Homeostasis in Late-Preterm and Term Infants. *Pediatrics* **2011**, *127*, 575–579. [CrossRef]
12. British Association of Perinatal Medicine. Identification and Management of Neonatal Hypoglycaemia in the Full Term Infant. Framework for Practice. *J. Hum. Lact.* **2017**, *35*, 521–523.
13. Mitanchez, D.H.-W.L.; Zimmermann, L.J.I.; Buonocore, G.; Beardsall, K.; Boardman, J.P.; Tin, W. Hypoglycaemia in at Risk Term Infants. 2018. Available online: https://www.efcni.org/wp-content/uploads/2023/05/2023_ESCNH_Standard_In_Brief_MEdicalCare.pdf (accessed on 20 June 2023).
14. Guidelines, Q.C. Hypoglycaemia–newborn. *Pediatr. Clin.* **2019**, *66*, 333–342.
15. Narvey, M.R.; Marks, S.D. The screening and management of newborns at risk for low blood glucose. *Paediatr. Child Health* **2019**, *24*, 536–544. [CrossRef]
16. Thornton, P.S.; Stanley, C.A.; De Leon, D.D.; Harris, D.; Haymond, M.W.; Hussain, K.; Levitsky, L.L.; Murad, M.H.; Rozance, P.J.; Simmons, R.A.; et al. Recommendations from the Pediatric Endocrine Society for Evaluation and Management of Persistent Hypoglycemia in Neonates, Infants, and Children. *J. Pediatr.* **2015**, *167*, 238–245. [CrossRef] [PubMed]
17. Güemes, M.; Rahman, S.A.; Hussain, K. What is a normal blood glucose? *Arch. Dis. Child.* **2016**, *101*, 569–574. [CrossRef] [PubMed]
18. Adam, P.A.J.; Räihä, N.; Rähialä, E.-L.; Kekomäki, M. Oxidation of glucose and D-B-OH-butyrate by the early human fetal brain. *Acta Paediatr. Scand.* **1975**, *64*, 17–24. [CrossRef] [PubMed]
19. Cornblath, M.; Reisner, S.H. Blood Glucose in the Neonate and Its Clinical Significance. *N. Engl. J. Med.* **1965**, *273*, 378–381. [CrossRef]
20. Stanley, C.A.; Rozance, P.J.; Thornton, P.S.; De Leon, D.D.; Harris, D.; Haymond, M.W.; Hussain, K.; Levitsky, L.L.; Murad, M.H.; Simmons, R.A.; et al. Re-Evaluating "Transitional Neonatal Hypoglycemia": Mechanism and Implications for Management. *J. Pediatr.* **2015**, *166*, 1520–1525.e1. [CrossRef]
21. Nicholl, R. What is the normal range of blood glucose concentrations in healthy term newborns? *Arch. Dis. Child.* **2003**, *88*, 238–239. [CrossRef]
22. Sinclair, J.C. Approaches to the definition of neonatal hypoglycemia. *Acta Paediatr. Jpn. Overseas Ed.* **1997**, *39*, S17–S20.
23. Rozance, P.J.; Hay, W.W. Hypoglycemia in Newborn Infants: Features Associated with Adverse Outcomes. *Neonatology* **2006**, *90*, 74–86. [CrossRef]
24. Hume, R.; McGeechan, A.; Burchell, A. Failure to detect preterm infants at risk of hypoglycemia before discharge. *J. Pediatr.* **1999**, *134*, 499–502. [CrossRef] [PubMed]
25. Holtrop, P.C. The Frequency of Hypoglycemia in Full-Term Large and Small for Gestational Age Newborns. *Am. J. Perinatol.* **1993**, *10*, 150–154. [CrossRef] [PubMed]
26. Agrawal, R.; Lui, K.; Gupta, J. Neonatal hypoglycaemia in infants of diabetic mothers. *J. Paediatr. Child Health* **2000**, *36*, 354–356. [CrossRef]
27. Hay, W.W.; Raju, T.N.; Higgins, R.D.; Kalhan, S.C.; Devaskar, S.U. Knowledge Gaps and Research Needs for Understanding and Treating Neonatal Hypoglycemia: Workshop Report from Eunice Kennedy Shriver National Institute of Child Health and Human Development. *J. Pediatr.* **2009**, *155*, 612–617. [CrossRef]
28. Diwakar, K.K.; Sasidhar, M.V. Plasma glucose levels in term infants who are appropriate size for gestation and exclusively breast fed. *Arch. Dis. Child.-Fetal Neonatal Ed.* **2002**, *87*, 46F–48F. [CrossRef]
29. Harding, J.E.; Harris, D.L.; Hegarty, J.E.; Alsweiler, J.M.; McKinlay, C.J. An emerging evidence base for the management of neonatal hypoglycaemia. *Early Hum. Dev.* **2016**, *104*, 51–56. [CrossRef]
30. Marcus, C. How to measure and interpret glucose in neonates. *Acta Paediatr.* **2001**, *90*, 963–964. [CrossRef]
31. Hussain, K.; Sharief, N. The inaccuracy of venous and capillary blood glucose measurement using reagent strips in the newborn period and the effect of haematocrit. *Early Hum. Dev.* **2000**, *57*, 111–121. [CrossRef]
32. Inoue, S.; Egi, M.; Kotani, J.; Morita, K. Accuracy of blood-glucose measurements using glucose meters and arterial blood gas analyzers in critically ill adult patients: Systematic review. *Crit. Care* **2013**, *17*, R48. [CrossRef] [PubMed]

33. Ge, X.; Lam, H.; Modi, S.J.; LaCourse, W.R.; Rao, G.; Tolosa, L. Comparing the Performance of the Optical Glucose Assay Based on Glucose Binding Protein with High-Performance Anion-Exchange Chromatography with Pulsed Electrochemical Detection: Efforts to Design a Low-Cost Point-of-Care Glucose Sensor. *J. Diabetes Sci. Technol.* **2007**, *1*, 864–872. [CrossRef]
34. McInerney, C.M.; Gupta, A. Delaying the First Bath Decreases the Incidence of Neonatal Hypoglycemia. *J. Obstet. Gynecol. Neonatal Nurs.* **2015**, *44*, S73–S74. [CrossRef]
35. Stomnaroska-Damcevski, O.; Petkovska, E.; Jancevska, S.; Danilovski, D. Neonatal Hypoglycemia: A Continuing Debate in Definition and Management. *Prilozi* **2015**, *36*, 91–97. [CrossRef] [PubMed]
36. Deshpande, S.; Platt, M.W. The investigation and management of neonatal hypoglycaemia. *Semin. Fetal Neonatal Med.* **2005**, *10*, 351–361. [CrossRef] [PubMed]
37. Hawdon, J.M.; Platt, M.P.W.; Aynsley-Green, A. Prevention and management of neonatal hypoglycaemia. *Arch. Dis. Child.-Fetal Neonatal Ed.* **1994**, *70*, F60–F65. [CrossRef]
38. Kalhan, S.; Peter-Wohl, S. Hypoglycemia: What is it for the neonate? *Am. J. Perinatol.* **2000**, *17*, 11–18. [CrossRef]
39. Harris, D.L.; Weston, P.J.; Signal, M.; Chase, J.G.; Harding, J.E. Dextrose gel for neonatal hypoglycaemia (the Sugar Babies Study): A randomised, double-blind, placebo-controlled trial. *Lancet* **2013**, *382*, 2077–2083. [CrossRef]
40. Harris, D.L.; Gamble, G.D.; Weston, P.J.; Harding, J.E. What Happens to Blood Glucose Concentrations After Oral Treatment for Neonatal Hypoglycemia? *J. Pediatr.* **2017**, *190*, 136–141. [CrossRef]
41. Auer, R.N.; Siesjö, B.K. Hypoglycaemia: Brain neurochemistry and neuropathology. *Baillieres Clin. Endocrinol. Metab.* **1993**, *7*, 611–625.
42. Hussain, K. Investigations for neonatal hypoglycaemia. *Clin. Biochem.* **2011**, *44*, 465–466. [CrossRef]
43. Lilien, L.D.; Pildes, R.S.; Srinivasan, G.; Voora, S.; Yeh, T.F. Treatment of neonatal hypoglycemia with minibolus and intraveous glucose infusion. *J. Pediatr.* **1980**, *7*, 295–298. [CrossRef]
44. Vanhatalo, T.; Tammela, O. Glucose infusions into peripheral veins in the management of neonatal hypoglycemia–20% instead of 15%? *Acta Paediatr.* **2010**, *99*, 350–353. [CrossRef] [PubMed]
45. Weston, P.J.; Harris, D.L.; Battin, M.; Brown, J.; Hegarty, J.E.; Harding, J.E. Oral dextrose gel for the treatment of hypoglycaemia in newborn infants. *Cochrane Database Syst. Rev.* **2016**, *5*, CD011027. [CrossRef] [PubMed]
46. Menni, F.; de Lonlay, P.; Sevin, C.; Touati, G.; Peigné, C.; Barbier, V.; Nihoul-Fékété, C.; Saudubray, J.-M.; Robert, J.-J. Neurologic Outcomes of 90 Neonates and Infants with Persistent Hyperinsulinemic Hypoglycemia. *Pediatrics* **2001**, *107*, 476–479. [CrossRef] [PubMed]
47. Burridge, N.; Symons, K. *Australian Injectable Drugs Handbook*, 7th ed.; Society of Hospital Pharmacists of Australia: Collingwood, Australia, 2017.
48. Rennie, J.M. *Roberton's Textbook of Neonatology*, 4th ed.; Elsevier Churchill Livingstone: Philadelphia, PA, USA, 2005.
49. Cloherty, J.P. *Manual of Neonatal Care*; Wolters Kluwer Health/Lippincott Williams & Wilkins: Philadelphia, PA, USA, 2012.

children

MDPI

Article

Understanding the Family Context: A Qualitative Descriptive Study of Parent and NICU Clinician Experiences and Perspectives

Maya Dahan [1,2,*], Leahora Rotteau [3], Shelley Higazi [2], Ophelia Kwayke [2], Giselle Lai [2], Wendy Moulsdale [2], Lisa Sampson [2], Jennifer Stannard [2], Paige Terrien Church [1,2] and Karel O'Brien [1,4]

1 Department of Pediatrics, Division of Neonatal-Perinatal Medicine, University of Toronto, Toronto, ON M5S, Canada
2 DAN Women & Babies Program, Department of Newborn and Developmental Pediatrics, Sunnybrook Health Sciences Centre, Toronto, ON M4N 3M5, Canada
3 Centre for Quality and Patient Safety, University of Toronto, Toronto, ON M5S, Canada
4 Department of Pediatrics, Mount Sinai Hospital, Sinai Health System, Toronto, ON M5G 1X5, Canada
* Correspondence: maya.dahan@sunnybrook.ca

Abstract: Enabling individualized decision-making for patients requires an understanding of the family context (FC) by healthcare providers. The FC is everything that makes the family unique, from their names, preferred pronouns, family structure, cultural or religious beliefs, and family values. While there is an array of approaches for individual clinicians to incorporate the FC into practice, there is a paucity of literature guiding the process of collecting and integrating the FC into clinical care by multidisciplinary interprofessional teams. The purpose of this qualitative study is to explore the experience of families and Neonatal Intensive Care Unit (NICU) clinicians with information sharing around the FC. Our findings illustrate that there are parallel and overlapping experiences of sharing the FC for families and clinicians. Both groups describe the positive impact of sharing the FC on building and sustaining relationships and on personalization of care and personhood. The experience by families of revolving clinicians and the risks of miscommunication about the FC were noted as challenges to sharing the FC. Parents described the desire to control the narrative about their FC, while clinicians described seeking equal access to the FC to support the family in the best way possible related to their clinical role. Our study highlights how the quality of care is positively impacted by clinicians' appreciation of the FC and the complex relationship between a large multidisciplinary interprofessional team and the family in an intensive care unit, while also highlighting the difficulties in its practical application. Knowledge learned can be utilized to inform the development of processes to improve communication between families and clinicians.

Keywords: communication; neonatology; family context; decision making

1. Introduction

In the late 20th century, decision-making in neonatology and in the wider medical field shifted from a paternalistic model, in which physicians make decisions regarding care for patients and families, towards a model guided by recognition of patient autonomy [1,2]. The latter model established a professional standard of providing detailed information about possible outcomes with the goal of allowing families to make independent 'informed decisions' [3,4]. However, research in psychology and behavioural economics has shown that data-guided parental choice is not categorical and bias-free [3,5]. Cognitive biases (such as framing effects, availability biases, commission bias, etc.) are omnipresent, especially in conversations with families [5–8]. Research has also highlighted that individuals make decisions based on their own lived experiences and values [9–12]. The pendulum has therefore swung back to the middle, to the intermediary between the decision-making spectrum extremes: a shared decision-making (SDM) model [12–15]. The SDM model, however, is not without its critics [16,17]. While the ideal model may remain debated, the need to understand a family's context (FC) is well agreed upon to be a crucial first step in building a relationship to facilitate decision-making with families [12,18,19]. The FC is everything that makes the family unique, from their names, preferred pronouns, family structure, and cultural or religious beliefs, to family values.

Positive impacts of learning about and sharing the FC have included facilitating clinicians' ability to have a holistic mindset [20] and to personalize care [12]. Contextualization of care, defined as adapting the medical plan to the patient's life context, or in the case of a neonate, the family's context, is a key competency for physicians [21,22]. There is an array of approaches for the individual clinician, often the physician, to collect and incorporate the FC into practice [12,18,23–25]; yet, there is no literature guiding the process of collecting and integrating FC into clinical care provided by a multidisciplinary interprofessional team.

The purpose of this descriptive qualitative study is to explore the experience of families and Neonatal Intensive Care Unit (NICU) clinicians with information sharing around the FC. We aim to further the understanding within the literature of how the quality of care is impacted by clinicians' appreciation of the FC and the complex relationship between a large multidisciplinary interprofessional team and the family in an intensive care unit setting. Understanding this issue from the perspective of families and clinicians is the critical first step to improving care [26,27]. Knowledge gained with this practice may then be utilized to inform the development of quality improvement (QI) processes aimed at improving communication between families and clinicians.

2. Methods

We conducted a descriptive qualitative study in a 42-bed tertiary care neonatal unit in Toronto, Canada, that cares for inborn and outborn infants requiring tertiary neonatal care. Patients reflect the broad multicultural and multilingual diversity of the City of Toronto.

Using purposive sampling, we sought maximum variation by selecting families with varying cultural backgrounds and educational levels and clinicians with varying professions, cultural backgrounds, and experience, were recruited [28]. Recruitment was stopped for each group when thematic saturation was reached [29].

This study was reviewed and approved by the Research Ethics Board of Sunnybrook Health Sciences Center. Each participant consented to participation. Semi-structured interviews were used to collect similar information from the participants while allowing personal stories and new concepts to emerge [30]. They occurred between August and December 2021. Interviews with the families were conducted by a physician (MD), and interviews with the clinicians were conducted by a research assistant with no prior relationship to the NICU or its staff. Semi-structured interview guides were used to lead the interviews and were modified in response to an iterative analysis. The development of the guides was informed by a review of the literature. The guides were piloted with an unrelated participant. They broadly focused on what participants shared about the FC, their experience of sharing the FC, and the decisions around how and when to share information about the FC [31]. The guides are available in Appendices A and B [31]. Interviews were transcribed using artificial intelligence and corrected and anonymized by the lead researcher (MD).

A thematic analysis was performed on the interview transcripts [32]. Two authors (MD + LR) read the first four transcripts for both groups (families and clinicians) and performed a preliminary analysis to generate a coding structure. The coding structure was then used by MD to code the remainder of the transcripts. The two lead researchers held regular analytic meetings following the steps for thematic analysis outlined by Braun and Clarke [33]. Through coding and analysis, we identified, defined, and named two important themes related to the experience of sharing the FC: the process of sharing the FC and the impact of sharing the FC. The two themes were examined for how they were similar and different among and between the parents and clinician groups.

The lead researcher (MD) was a neonatal fellow working at the institution. Although there was a degree of involvement in the care of the patients whose families were interviewed during on-call shifts, MD was not a member of their core clinical team. The second researcher (LR) held solely a research role and was not part of the neonatal care team. The remainder of the research team was part of the multidisciplinary interprofessional team at the research site. The research team helped formulate the project details and provided feedback on the interview guide as well as a review of this manuscript.

3. Results

3.1. Demographic of Participants

Eleven parents making up eight families were interviewed (Table 1). One parent removed themselves from the study after the interview was completed; their interview was not included in the analysis. All parents had infants who were born at less than 29 weeks of gestation and with birthweights less than 1000 g. Infants were 3–14 weeks old at the time of the interviews. Four of the ten participants' first language was not English. Eleven clinicians from varying disciplines were interviewed (Table 2).

Table 1. Demographics of Families.

Fictitious Name	Gender	Marital Status	Other Children	Self-Identified Ethnicity	English as Mother Tongue	Highest Level of Education	Child's Gestational Age *
Chloe	Female	Married	None	White	Yes	PhD	26–27 weeks
George	Male	Married	None	White	Yes	PhD	26–27 weeks
Sanjeeva	Male	Married	None	South Asian	No	University	24–25 weeks
Chandan	Female	Married	None	South Asian	No	University	24–25 weeks
Zain	Male	Common law	None	Black	No	Trade certificate	24–25 weeks
Bianca	Female	Common law	None	Black	Yes	High school	24–25 weeks
Simi	Female	Married	2+ other children	Black	Yes	College	28–29 weeks
Marie	Female	Single	None	Black	Yes	University diploma	22–23 weeks
Shaden	Female	Married	1 other child	Arab, South Asian	Yes	University—above bachelor	22–23 weeks
Sarah	Female	Common law	None	Black	No	Bachelor's degree	26–27 weeks

* GA reported as a range to preserve anonymity.

Table 2. Demographics of Clinicians.

Discipline	Number of Participants
Neonatologist	3
Nursing team leader	3
Nurse practitioner	3
Social worker	1
Respiratory therapist	1

3.2. Thematic Analysis

Two interconnected overarching themes were identified in both the family and clinician interviews: *the process* and *the impact* of sharing information about a family's context (FC). Figure 1 shows the parallel between the two themes and their subthemes as experienced by both families and clinicians.

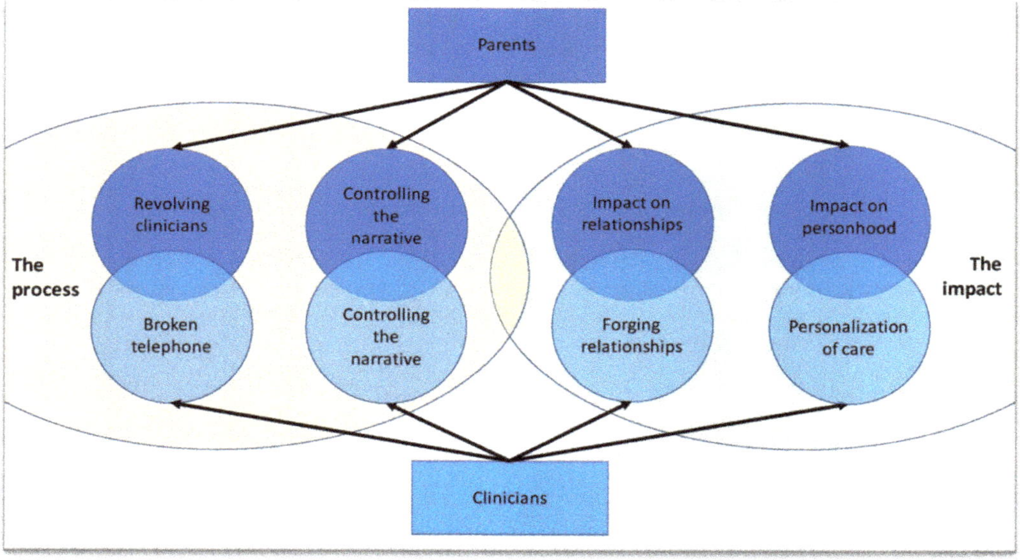

Figure 1. Venn diagrams visually depicting the relationship between two overarching themes and their subthemes. It highlights the parallels and overlapping experiences of the families with those of the clinicians.

3.2.1. Process

The first theme describes the process by which families shared information about their FC with clinicians and the process by which clinicians shared information about FC with the other members of the care team.

3.2.2. The Process: Family Perspective

In the following section, the family perspective of the process is presented using two subthemes: *revolving clinicians*, which describes the process of information sharing as seen by families and how they experienced it, and *controlling the narrative*, describing parents' underlying desire to control the narrative about their context.

3.3. *Revolving Clinicians*

Parents described a general openness to sharing information about themselves and their family, which, when asked, usually occurred informally at the bedside. When asked whom they shared information with, families invariably brought up the seemingly endless revolving rotation of clinicians. George explains:

> *"There's people coming in and out all the time, and you have one doctor on Saturday morning, and you never see them again, there's another doctor on Saturday night, you never see them again [...] you develop a sort of little relationship with someone and then you never see them again."*

With this perpetual change in providers, parents noticed a disconnection between providers related to the FC. George continued to describe the need to create *"an efficient narrative, otherwise you're just exhausted"* because of the constant need to reiterate this narrative to each new provider. Chandan emphasized this constant repetition *"if we had the consistency, then they already knew us. And they knew that, you know, they don't have to provide with the same information each and every day"*. Chloe worried that one day with *"fatigue setting in, we're just not going to give all the info [...] and then [the clinicians] won't get the whole story and they wouldn't be able to cater their treatment to our situation"*. The need for repetition was specific to the family context and did not include the infant's medical history. Parents described their experience of sharing information about their context as generally positive with individual clinicians but exhausting due to the repetition.

3.4. Controlling the Narrative

Parents had an underlying desire to control the narrative about their context, both its creation and its evolution. For example, Chloe preferred to be asked upfront questions about her context because it would make her *"feel like I would have control over the situation a little bit more"*, explaining she already felt a lack of control in their NICU journey. She was also initially skeptical about sharing information about her context, unclear about the *"tenor of the interaction [...] maybe it's a question of utility, like what is that information used for"*. Simi wanted clinicians to understand her busy home life with her four school-aged children. Similarly, Shaden felt *"it helps reduce the guilt when I have to leave [...] it's so much easier if people just know that bigger context, right?"* once the bedside nurses knew she picked up her son from school every day. Several of the parents described forging relationships with those caring for their child as they believed they would get even better care if clinicians *"remember [them], you know, just trying to keep [baby] on the map, even though I know it's their job. But just to me, it's like the one thing I can do is like, engage them in that way"* (George).

Shaden initially feared being stigmatized because of her appearance: *"I know that systemic biases exist, and don't know how it would necessarily play out here. That gap makes it scarier"*. As she was able to share more about her context and feel more understood, she described the fear dissipating. Her ability to share her FC increased her sense of personhood and reduced her feelings of stigmatization. Overall, families desired a sense of control over one of the few variables that was within reach when their infant is unexpectedly hospitalized in the NICU: their own family narrative.

The Process: Clinicians Perspective

In the following section, the process is described from the clinicians' perspective. When discussing the process for sharing information about the FC with clinicians, participants noted the importance of both sharing between families and clinicians and between clinicians. Two subthemes are outlined: *the broken telephone* and *controlling the narrative.*

3.5. The Broken Telephone

Clinicians described relying on verbal handover due to the inconsistency in written documentation about the FC. Though several clinicians commented on the potential risks of relying on verbal information sharing; *"if it's not written, it didn't happen. And that's how stories get made up"* (RN), they rarely reported looking at the patient chart to find this information. Finding information about the FC was difficult, due to sporadic documentation and the many possible locations to document within the electronic medical record (EMR). Throughout the interviews, 17 different locations were identified where information about the FC could be found, many of which were discipline-specific. A social worker, who regularly documented in the chart, expressed her frustration with this approach; *"people don't always read the chart [...] and so it all has to be repeated [...] that's not efficient, and it doesn't feel all that respectful"*.

Poorly written handover practices about the FC and the subsequent reliance on verbal handover created fertile ground for information disconnection described as a broken telephone. One nurse described this process: *"It's kind of like if somebody hears a story [...] especially juicy stories [...] a lot of it gets embellished as the story goes down the telephone line. So maybe things are kind of, exaggerated"*. Another nurse elaborated: *"What would happen is a rumor mill. Okay, it's not necessarily written down, but what people say may not be true, or they may have a different opinion or they've misunderstood something"*. A neonatologist gave examples of how this approach left room for biases:

> *"You're making assumptions about people based on something about their background. Teenage mothers, people who take drugs, cultural things sometimes, you know, so there's different reasons that I think we're either labeling or judging those sorts of things. That's not really positive."*

The 'broken telephone' was identified as a serious gap in their ability to care for patients, with potential detrimental effects on families.

3.6. Controlling the Narrative

Clinicians wanted equal access to the FC in order to better care for patients since *"the social and the medical needs to go together in order to better serve [families]"* (RN). However, many clinicians reported inconsistent access. A social worker explained how everyone wants to contribute to it in their own way, independent of their professional role:

> *"There are some practitioners, regardless of discipline, who make a point of trying to really learn about the family. And it doesn't mean that they're necessarily the ones sitting down and asking the family about their circumstances about their supports about mental health history about their understanding of the medical, you know, they're gathering it from colleagues, from other people's interactions with the family, from documentation in the chart."*

Each clinician articulated a goal to create their own relationship with the family but also an interest in furthering the relationship between the family and care team. In addition to providing better care, strong relationships also improved their own work experience. This desire to understand the FC was heightened in the more medically fragile infant. *"If the baby's critical [...], you might speak to them every day"*, said one of the neonatologists as they described the increased volume of interactions and the perception of a more imminent impact on the family and the baby. Clinicians did not seek to control the content of the family narrative the same way parents did; instead, they sought equal access to it to be able to support the family in the best way possible related to their clinical role.

4. The Impact

The second overarching theme describes the impact of sharing information about the FC for clinicians and families; specifically, the *impact on relationships* and the *respect of personhood*.

4.1. The Impact: Families Perspective

4.1.1. Impact on Relationships

Parents felt a connection and establishment of trust when clinicians demonstrated interest in the FC. They spoke of *"highly personalized information catered to us"* (Chloe) when the FC was well understood. As described above, parents experienced an improvement in care once they established relationships with clinicians. Shaden explained:

> *"It was so helpful because then everybody knew that we had another kid [...] It was a game changer. Like we got to do kangaroo care* (Kangaroo care is a method of holding a baby skin to skin) *so much more and I think it was just helpful for people to know that there was this other major piece that governed our interactions."*

She continued to elaborate on how it made a big difference when a nurse knew her context; it *"builds trust, like you really need that with this situation. Like, if you can't have a communication I don't know how you'd be able to leave your baby in the room and walk away"*. Marie spoke about how the ability to bond over commonality helped lessen her anxiety; *"the nurse basically said her son went through it and he played he started playing after surgery right after the next day so [...] okay, it's not gonna be that bad to do the surgery"*. Sarah described the emotional relief provided by an opportunity to speak about something other than her baby's day to day care: *"a little off the topic [but] I'm able to share excitement about my job [...] so I felt like it was it was good for me [...] even though the focus is on [baby] it gives me that break from my head"*. For Sanjeeva and Chandan, sharing their FC was the root of their relationships:

> *"It makes us feel more connected. And then we can share the thoughts with the nurses. And then that way, we develop a connection with the nurses as well, because they also understand where we come from, what we do, and then I would say, it develops in affection as well with the family."*

However, not every parent spontaneously shared their FC. Zain and Bianca, self-described as quiet and introverted people, worried they would be disliked if they overshared. They only shared when asked. When the door was opened for them to share their beliefs and values, it allowed for services to be provided that they otherwise would not have known about and also made them *"feel good that somebody wants to know what my beliefs are"* (Bianca).

4.1.2. Impact on Personhood

Taking the time to understand the FC was interpreted by parents as respecting their personhood. Parents spoke about the drastic turn their life took when they had a preterm child and appreciated when clinicians took the time to understand who they were as individuals. It made parents feel like the clinicians *"care about both my son and myself"* (Simi). Sarah elaborated on why this is important: *"Mom also needs to heal as much as baby needs to heal. So it's a good healing process for mom"*. Parents gave examples of how this respect for their personhood was displayed. For Bianca, it was the meticulous care for her necklace she had left in her baby's incubator and the books she had placed in the room; for Marie, it was showing interest in her business and getting updates on her family members; for Shaden, it was checking in about her mental health; for Zain, it was being offered the opportunity to share his religious and cultural views; and for George and Chloe, it was the opportunity to talk about their family values.

Taking the time to understand the FC fostered trust in the individual clinician but also had the ability to positively or negatively colour the relationship with the entire group represented by that single clinician (e.g., professional group, the unit within the hospital, etc.). George compared their experience in the NICU with their experience in the high-risk obstetrical unit despite only having met a few of the physicians in each unit:

> *"The doctors in the NICU have been more warm and more generous with their time than the doctors and OBs that we encountered in the floor up, the sort of labor birthing floor, I forget the names of those areas, but they were more sort of business. And sometimes they would just sort of talk to each other and ignore us, you know? And we're like, hey, like, we have a question or what's going on? Or what are you talking about? Or why is there a worry tone in your voice? And that's just not the case, in NICU, we've loved all the doctors there."*

Chandan compared primary nurses to all other nurses:

> *"I feel if they are primary, they feel like they own it, if they are not primary then why bother to know the baby or, it's more of an attitude with the baby. I don't have to know the baby, I am just here, I just have to take care of them and go."*

Bianca compared her experience in the NICU to her previous medical encounters, highlighting how being asked about her context was seen as a sign of respect: *"there are some doctors that don't even let you talk. Here, they ask what your culture is"*. However, she also reflected on how she initially hesitated to share, fearful of judgement based on her visible demographics. Hearing stories of *"some of the anti-black racism [or] the Islamophobia [...] especially when you're in such a vulnerable position, you're [...] worried that that's going to play a role"*. All of these examples speak to the nuances of how communication shaped the feeling of respect that is reflected upon an entire care team, as well as the hesitation parents may have to share.

4.2. The Impact: Clinicians Perspective

4.2.1. Personalization of Care

Clinicians overwhelmingly spoke about the positive impacts of understanding the FC, such as the increased ability to be respectful, empathetic, and accepting, allowing for a greater appreciation of the individuality of each family and a better ability to personalize care. A respiratory therapist (RT) spoke about discovering *"those special precious moments that they'll never get back"* that is of unique importance to certain families, but clinicians will only know if they ask. Another clinician elaborated: *"Some religions or cultures have certain practices that are time sensitive [...] so if we know what those are, we can help identify and have the resources available to us and to the families"* (NP). This is crucial in the care provided as *"the patient [...] is not alone. They exist within a family, a framework. And family doesn't just mean mum and dad, it can mean you know, a broader community"* (MD). Understanding the FC not only helped personalize what was offered to parents but also how clinicians approached communication.

> *"If a mom was raised with a sibling who had cerebral palsy, they are worried about different things, then a family who's got no medical background, and has never had a baby in the hospital. So their stressors are different. And how we help them cope can sometimes be different."* (NP)

This personalization afforded opportunities to adapt the approach to the individual family, anticipating and addressing their unique concerns.

> *"When we understand these things about families and their facilitators and barriers to being at the bedside and helping their children grow and develop, which we know is important [...], then we're better able to help them be present at the bedside."* (NP)

Sharing this type of information between clinicians helped *"the next person that's meeting the family [to] have a little bit more context as to where they're coming from and, and what might be important for them"* (NP). Ultimately, *"the more we know about the person, the family, them in their environment, them within this medical environment, what their needs are, their questions, I think, the better able we are to provide the care that we do"* (SW). Clinicians unanimously viewed this shared mental model as facilitating better care.

4.2.2. Forging Relationships

Beyond the ability to provide personalized and empathetic care for babies and families, understanding the FC also provided an opportunity for clinicians to forge relationships with the families. A nurse practitioner described that there is *"something that's kind of nice to be able be able to have a conversation with parents"* (NP) regarding life outside the NICU. It improved the sense of collaboration clinicians feel with families (MD), and all clinician participants reflected positively on their experience of caring for families with whom they were able to further their relationship by understanding their FC. However, in the context of the busy NICU environment, several clinicians reflected upon concerns regarding the time commitment to collect and share information on the FC.

5. Discussion

The present study described how families and clinicians experienced sharing information about the FC. The impact of knowing and sharing this information was positively described by all participants, but the process was highlighted as fragmented. The benefits of sharing the FC have been described across a range of settings including adult, pediatric, and neonatal units [6,12,18,20,21,24]. Our findings complement the existing literature by further exploring these impacts, specifically in the NICU setting. Sharing FC supports relationship building and personalization of care and provides an opportunity to respect the personhood of patients and families [34].

Study findings described how both clinicians and families identified a desire to control information about the FC. Control was perceived as enabling enhanced patient-centred care. However, families and clinicians seemed to have different motivations for controlling the narrative. Families wanted control over *shaping* their narrative and how they were perceived, while clinicians wanted ease of *access* to the narrative to better support their patients. A similar theme was found in the literature under the umbrella of narrative competence. Narrative competence is defined as "the set of skills required to recognize, absorb, interpret, and be moved by the stories one hears or reads" [35]. Narrative competence helps clinicians and families engage with each other not only in the patient–clinician relationship but also in the human–human relationship, improving the experience for all those involved [36,37]. The theme described by our participants showed a desire to use the family context as a means of building a relationship between parents and clinicians to improve care.

While families and clinicians alike discussed this shared goal in the interviews, they also spoke about the skills and the infrastructure needed to facilitate narrative competence in the NICU setting [34]. Key to achieving the goal of relationship building is *the process* by which information about the FC gets shared by families and between clinicians and the perceived enablers and barriers. Parents and clinicians described how the process varied between individual clinicians and referred to the broken telephone and fragmentation that occurred due to the revolving door of clinicians involved in each infant's care throughout their long journey in the NICU.

Beyond the lack of infrastructure to support sharing the FC, participants in our study also alluded to the perceived pitfalls of integrating FC into care. Clinicians worry about the time required to understand the FC. Some parents in our study hesitated to share their FC because of the fear of being stigmatized based on their context. Concerns in the literature also centred on the time necessary to understand a patient's context, the education, and the culture shift necessary for its success [38,39]. Interestingly, while people worry about being stigmatized, it is argued that the antidote to this stigma, founded in implicit bias, is actually contextualizing care [40].

Our findings highlight the variability in clinician communication skills and documentation, leading to the reliance on verbal handover, which is fraught with the risk of inaccuracies and misinterpretation. Though certain clinicians felt that understanding the FC would help them provide more narratively competent care, they did not know whether this information was ever collected by their colleagues, or if so, where to find it within the patient chart. We found that sharing the FC often relied on verbal handover. Similar to unstructured verbal handover of clinical information, reliance on verbal handover of FC risks the omission of important details, unnecessary inclusion of superfluous information, and the 'broken telephone' phenomenon [41]. Through the interviews, we discovered that information about the FC was being documented in 17 different places within the medical record. Participants described how this inconsistency can lead to miscommunication and gossip, requiring families to repeat themselves or correct misinformation. Clinician participants also described the complexities of handover within a large multidisciplinary interprofessional team, highlighting an area for improvement in the care of neonates and their families.

Fragmentation of communication is a problem that has been described before in terms of relationships and experiences of care [41], which can be addressed with the standardization of various processes across care providers, development of guidelines, communication tools, standardized order sets, and checklists [42–47]. Similar approaches can potentially be applied and adapted to communication about the FC but require further exploration to ensure an appropriate balance between the standardization of the approach to collection and documentation while still promoting the personalization of information.

Despite these technical challenges highlighted by participants, findings from the interviews for both clinicians and families highlight the importance of consistency in care providers during the often lengthy NICU stay. Consistency led to a better understanding of the FC, which in turn resulted in building trusting relationships; it is these relationships that lessened parental anxiety.

Our study has limitations. Firstly, only parents who felt comfortable being interviewed in English were included. While families that did not speak English well enough to participate in an interview are likely to have had a different experience based on the ease of communication, English was a second language for almost half of our participants. Secondly, we only interviewed families and clinicians about their experiences, we did not observe them interacting. Additionally, this was a single-site study and focused on the NICU. While a focus on the uniqueness of the NICU setting allowed further depth and a better understanding of the intricate dynamics that exist within the team, this may limit the generalizability to other settings. A strength of our study was that we interviewed clinicians with varying backgrounds professionally and culturally. Moreover, the use of qualitative methods facilitated a deeper exploration of the process the team used to understand the FC as well as the nuances in the impact of knowing the family context had on the care provided.

6. Conclusions

Results of this descriptive qualitative study emphasize the vastly positive impacts of sharing the FC on the care provided to infants and their families in the NICU, while also highlighting the difficulties in the practical application of this practice. It furthers the understanding within the literature of the impact of integrating the FC on care experiences and the complex relationship between a large, multidisciplinary, interprofessional team and the family in an intensive care unit. Armed with this knowledge, a targeted approach can be created to improve the current process by addressing gaps highlighted by families and clinicians and focusing on the positive impacts described. Beyond the implementation of a tool or a checklist, family context needs to be integrated into each aspect of clinical care to facilitate the narrative competence desired by families and clinicians alike.

Author Contributions: Conceptualization, M.D., L.R., S.H., O.K., G.L., W.M., L.S., J.S., P.T.C. and K.O.; data curation, M.D., P.T.C. and K.O.; formal analysis, M.D., L.R., P.T.C. and K.O.; funding acquisition, M.D., P.T.C. and K.O.; investigation, M.D., L.R., P.T.C. and K.O.; methodology, M.D., L.R., P.T.C. and K.O.; project administration, M.D. and P.T.C.; resources, M.D.; supervision, P.T.C. and K.O.; validation, M.D., L.R., P.T.C. and K.O.; visualization, M.D., L.R., S.H., O.K., G.L., W.M., L.S., J.S., P.T.C. and K.O.; writing—original draft, M.D. and L.R.; writing—review and editing, L.R., S.H., O.K., G.L., W.M., L.S., J.S., P.T.C. and K.O. All authors have read and agreed to the published version of the manuscript.

Funding: This study was partially funded by CHILD-BRIGHT Graduate Student Fellowship in Patient-oriented Research.

Institutional Review Board Statement: The study approved by the Institutional Review Board of Sunnybrook Health Sciences Centre on 9 July 2021, reference number 3775.

Informed Consent Statement: Informed consent was obtained from all subjects involved in the study.

Data Availability Statement: The data presented in this study are available on request from the corresponding author. The data are not publicly available due to it being qualitative data and can breach patient confidentiality.

Acknowledgments: Thank you to Farah Tahsin for her help with the clinician interviews, Laura Borges for her help organizing interviews, the parents and clinicians who participated in the interviews, and the NICU Sunnybrook team.

Conflicts of Interest: The authors declare no conflict of interest.

Appendix A

Semi-structured interviews with parents:

Preamble

Thank you so much for meeting with me today and agreeing to participate in this interview. I want to remind you that what you say here is confidential and will not be linked back to you or your child, or identify you in any way. I am recording this interview so that I can transcribe it. This means I will type out the words said in this interview into a secure document for analysis. There will be no identifiers on the transcripts. The de-identified transcripts will be accessed by other members of the research team to perform the analysis.

The purpose of this interview is to explore your experiences and perceptions of your medical team in understanding of who you are as a family. We are trying to understand *how* they can get that information in a way that works both for you, your child and the medical team. We are here to learn from you, so anything you have to share is welcomed. Nothing you say here will affect in any way the care your child receives. There are no right or wrong answers.

Questions:

1. Would you be able to describe to me your family structure and what is most important to you as a family?
2. Can you please share with me what your experience sharing information with staff in the NICU has been like?
3. Can you share with me any instances where you shared with members of the medical team information this information?
    a. Can you share some examples?
    b. Can you describe where these conversations took place?
    c. Can you describe why you shared that information?
    d. Can you share with me your thoughts about how the information was collected and your perspective on being respected as a parent during these conversations?
    e. Were there instances where you felt more comfortable having these conversations than others? Can you say more about this?
    f. Can you recal any instances where you have had to repeat this information several times to the members of the medical team? Can you describe these? How did it make you feel?
4. Can you share with me any factors that you felt affected your ability or desire to share this information? I will use some prompts to help you think about this.
    a. I am curious about any personal factors that affected your ability to share this information? (ex. Cultural or language barriers, the acuity of your child's illness)
    b. I am curious about any enviornmental factor that affected your ability to share this information? (ex. Timing, location)
    c. I am curious about any specific things about the person asking you these questions that affected your ability to share this information? (ex. Their role, gender, culture etc.
5. How did sharing this information affect the care you received? Can you say more about this?
    a. Can you describe how this information was used?
    b. Do you feel that this information was used appropriately? If so, why? If not, why not?
6. Babies in the NICU are cared for by a large team of people. The medical team shares information about patients to facilitate care between team members. Can you share with me your thoughts on how this information about your family was shared between the different members of the medical team during your hospital stay?
    a. What made you feel like it was or wasn't shared? Could you say more about this?
    b. How did that make you feel?
    c. What do you think the medical team could do better?
7. Overall, do you feel the medical team or members of the medical team have a good sense of who your family is and what is important to you? Can you describe why or why not?
8. How would it make you feel if staff asked a standardized list of questions to collect this information?
    a. How would it make you feel if other members of the team referred to this information?

Wrap-up

We really appreciate your time and insights. Before we wrap up, is there anything that you think is important for us to know about how the NICU staff communicate with families and learn what is important to them?

If I realized I missed anything when I review our conversation, would it be okay if I follow up with you by phone or email?

Appendix B

Clinician semi-structured interviews

Preamble

Thank you so much for meeting with me today and agreeing to participate in this interview. Just to remind you that everything you say here is confidential and will not be linked back to you or identify you in any way. I am recording this interview so that I can transcribe it. The interview will be transcribed and there will be no identifiers on the transcripts. The other members of the research team will only access the de-identified transcripts to perform the analysis.

The purpose of this interview is to better understand what you think about *how* the medical team learns about the social and cultural circumstances of families and what is important to them. We would also like to understand what you think about *how* the medical team uses this information in their communication with families. We are here to learn from you, so anything you have to share is welcome. There are no right or wrong answers.

Questions

1. In your experience, what are the key pieces of information that are most valuable to you in caring for a patient and understanding the family context?
2. How would you describe the way or ways you get information about a family and what is important to them?
    a. Can you describe the setting in which you get this information from families?
    b. Can you describe the process of sharing this information with other team members?
    c. Can you describe the process of getting this information from other team members?
3. Can you share with me any factors that you feel affect your ability to collect this information? I will provide you some prompts to think about this.
    a. Can you describe any patient factors that might influence this? (ex. Cultural or language barriers, patient acuity)
    b. Can you describe any enviornmental factors that might influence this ? (ex. Timing, location)
    c. Can you describe any equipement factors that might influence this? (ex lack of resources, lack of tools)
    d. Can you describe any medical team factors that might influence this? (ex. Cultural, hierarchical, educational)
4. Can you describe your ideal way of collecting this information?
5. Can you describe how this information about families is typically handed over between members of the medical team?
    a. Can you reflect on some of the positives of this process? What about some of the negatives of this process?
    b. How does this process make you feel?
6. How do you feel like this information is being considered when interacting with families? Please elaborate.
    a. How do you think this is done well?
    b. How do you think it could be improved?
7. Why do you feel this information should be considered when interacting with families?

8. What do you think works well in our current process of collecting and sharing information about a family's context and what is important to them? Please elaborate.
9. What do you think doesn't work well in our current process? Please elaborate.
10. How would it make you feel to have a standardized form to guide collection of this information?
    a. How would it make you feel to obtain some of this information from a standardized form when it has been gathered by others?

Wrap-up

We really appreciate your time and insights. Before we wrap up, is there anything else that you think is important for us to know about the tools and processes used to support communication between families and the medical staff in the NICU.

If I realized I missed anything when I review our conversation, would it be okay if I follow up with you by phone or email?

References

1. Sullivan, A.; Cummings, C. Historical Perspectives: Shared Decision Making in the NICU. *Neoreviews* **2020**, *21*, e217–e225. [CrossRef] [PubMed]
2. Emanuel, E.J.; Emanuel, L.L. Four models of the physician-patient relationship. *JAMA* **1992**, *267*, 2221–2226. [CrossRef] [PubMed]
3. Lantos, J.D. Ethical Problems in Decision Making in the Neonatal ICU. *N. Engl. J. Med.* **2018**, *379*, 1851–1860. [CrossRef] [PubMed]
4. Ward, F.R. Parents and professionals in the NICU: Communication within the context of ethical decision making—An integrative review. *Neonatal Netw.* **2005**, *24*, 25–33. [CrossRef]
5. Sisk, B.A.; Baker, J.N. Microethics of Communication-Hidden Roles of Bias and Heuristics in the Words We Choose. *JAMA Pediatr.* **2018**, *172*, 1115–1116. [CrossRef]
6. Ubel, P.A.; Scherr, K.A.; Fagerlin, A. Empowerment Failure: How Shortcomings in Physician Communication Unwittingly Undermine Patient Autonomy. *Am. J. Bioeth.* **2017**, *17*, 31–39. [CrossRef]
7. Dahan, M.; Banihani, R.; Church, P.T. Neonatal research outcomes: The ethical imperative to change attitudes. *Lancet Child Adolesc. Health* **2022**, *6*, 449–450. [CrossRef]
8. Haward, M.; Mercurio, M.; Janvier, A. Perpetuating Biases and Injustice Toward Preterm Infants. *Am. J. Bioeth.* **2017**, *17*, 27–29. [CrossRef]
9. Tversky, A.; Kahneman, D. The Framing of Decisions and the Psychology of Choice. *Science* **1981**, *211*, 453–458. [CrossRef]
10. Carling, C.L.; Kristoffersen, D.T.; Montori, V.M.; Herrin, J.; Schünemann, H.J.; Treweek, S.; Akl, E.A.; Oxman, A.D. The effect of alternative summary statistics for communicating risk reduction on decisions about taking statins: A randomized trial. *PLoS Med.* **2009**, *6*, e1000134. [CrossRef]
11. Carling, C.L.; Kristoffersen, D.T.; Flottorp, S.; Fretheim, A.; Oxman, A.D.; Schünemann, H.J.; Akl, E.A.; Herrin, J.; MacKenzie, T.D.; Montori, V.M. The effect of alternative graphical displays used to present the benefits of antibiotics for sore throat on decisions about whether to seek treatment: A randomized trial. *PLoS Med.* **2009**, *6*, e1000140. [CrossRef]
12. Kukora, S.K.; Boss, R.D. Values-based shared decision-making in the antenatal period. *Semin. Fetal Neonatal Med.* **2018**, *23*, 17–24. [CrossRef]
13. Soltys, F.; Philpott-Streiff, S.E.; Fuzzell, L.; Politi, M.C. The importance of shared decision-making in the neonatal intensive care unit. *J. Perinatol.* **2020**, *40*, 504–509. [CrossRef]
14. Kalsi, D.; Ward, J.; Lee, R.; Fulford, K.; Handa, A. Shared decision-making across the specialties: Much potential but many challenges. *J. Eval. Clin. Pract.* **2019**, *25*, 1050–1054. [CrossRef]
15. Forum, N.Q. *NQP Shared Decision Making Action Brief*; National Quality Forum: Washington, DC, USA, 2017.
16. Coulter, A. Partnerships with patients: The pros and cons of shared clinical decision-making. *J. Health Serv. Res. Policy* **1997**, *2*, 112–121. [CrossRef]
17. Geurtzen, R.; Draaisma, J.; Hermens, R.; Scheepers, H.; Woiski, M.; van Heijst, A.; Hogeveen, M. Various experiences and preferences of Dutch parents in prenatal counseling in extreme prematurity. *Patient Educ. Couns.* **2018**, *101*, 2179–2185. [CrossRef]
18. Haward, M.F.; Gaucher, N.; Payot, A.; Robson, K.; Janvier, A. Personalized Decision Making: Practical Recommendations for Antenatal Counseling for Fragile Neonates. *Clin. Perinatol.* **2017**, *44*, 429–445. [CrossRef]
19. Klawetter, S.; Cetin, N.; Ilea, P.; McEvoy, C.; Dukhovny, D.; Saxton, S.N.; Rincon, M.; Rodriguez-JenKins, J.; Nicolaidis, C. "All these people saved her life, but she needs me too": Understanding and responding to parental mental health in the NICU. *J. Perinatol.* **2022**, *42*, 1496–1503. [CrossRef]
20. Orkin, J.; Beaune, L.; Moore, C.; Weiser, N.; Arje, D.; Rapoport, A.; Netten, K.; Adams, S.; Cohen, E.; Amin, R. Toward an Understanding of Advance Care Planning in Children with Medical Complexity. *Pediatrics* **2020**, *145*, e20192241. [CrossRef]
21. Weiner, S.J. Contextualizing care: An essential and measurable clinical competency. *Patient Educ. Couns.* **2022**, *105*, 594–598. [CrossRef]

22. Schwartz, A.; Weiner, S.J.; Binns-Calvey, A.; Weaver, F.M. Providers contextualise care more often when they discover patient context by asking: Meta-analysis of three primary data sets. *BMJ Qual. Saf.* **2016**, *25*, 159–163. [CrossRef] [PubMed]
23. Franck, L.S.; Waddington, C.; O'Brien, K. Family Integrated Care for Preterm Infants. *Crit. Care Nurs. Clin. N. Am.* **2020**, *32*, 149–165. [CrossRef] [PubMed]
24. Lantos, J.D. What Is the Purpose of Antenatal Counseling? *J. Pediatr.* **2018**, *196*, 8–10. [CrossRef] [PubMed]
25. Lemyre, B.; Moore, G. Counselling and management for anticipated extremely preterm birth. *Paediatr. Child Health* **2017**, *22*, 334–341. [CrossRef]
26. Booth, A.; Noyes, J.; Flemming, K.; Moore, G.; Tunçalp, Ö.; Shakibazadeh, E. Formulating questions to explore complex interventions within qualitative evidence synthesis. *BMJ Glob. Health* **2019**, *4*, e001107. [CrossRef]
27. Robert, G.; Cornwell, J.; Locock, L.; Purushotham, A.; Sturmey, G.; Gager, M. Patients and staff as codesigners of healthcare services. *BMJ* **2015**, *350*, g7714. [CrossRef]
28. Patton, M.Q. *Qualitative Research and Evaluation Methods*; Laughton, C.D., Ed.; Sage Publications, Inc.: Newbury Park, CA, USA, 2002.
29. Hennink, M.M.; Kaiser, B.N.; Marconi, V.C. Code Saturation Versus Meaning Saturation: How Many Interviews Are Enough? *Qual. Health Res.* **2017**, *27*, 591–608. [CrossRef]
30. Brinkmann, S. Unstructured and Semi-Structured Interviewing. In *The Oxford Handbook of Qualitative Research*; Leavy, P., Ed.; Oxford University Press: Cary, NC, USA, 2014; pp. 277–299.
31. Kallio, H.; Pietilä, A.M.; Johnson, M.; Kangasniemi, M. Systematic methodological review: Developing a framework for a qualitative semi-structured interview guide. *J. Adv. Nurs.* **2016**, *72*, 2954–2965. [CrossRef]
32. Terry, G.H.; Hayfield, N.; Clarke, V.; Braun, V. Thematic Analysis. In *The SAGE Handbook of Qualitative Research in Psychology*; Willig, C.R., Stainton, W., Eds.; SAGE Publications Ltd.: London, UK, 2017. [CrossRef]
33. Braun, V.; Clarke, V. *Successful Qualitative Research: A Practical Guide for Beginners*; SAGE Publications Inc.: London, UK, 2013.
34. Sigurdson, K.; Profit, J.; Dhurjati, R.; Morton, C.; Scala, M.; Vernon, L.; Randolph, A.; Phan, J.T.; Franck, L.S. Former NICU Families Describe Gaps in Family-Centered Care. *Qual. Health Res.* **2020**, *30*, 1861–1875. [CrossRef]
35. Charon, R. Narrative and medicine. *N. Engl. J. Med.* **2004**, *350*, 862–864. [CrossRef]
36. Charon, R. The patient-physician relationship. Narrative medicine: A model for empathy, reflection, profession, and trust. *JAMA* **2001**, *286*, 1897–1902. [CrossRef]
37. Zaharias, G. What is narrative-based medicine? Narrative-based medicine 1. *Can. Fam. Physician* **2018**, *64*, 176–180.
38. Kalitzkus, V.; Matthiessen, P.F. Narrative-based medicine: Potential, pitfalls, and practice. *Perm. J.* **2009**, *13*, 80–86. [CrossRef]
39. Schwartz, A.; Weiner, S.J.; Harris, I.B.; Binns-Calvey, A. An Educational Intervention for Contextualizing Patient Care and Medical Students' Abilities to Probe for Contextual Issues in Simulated Patients. *JAMA* **2010**, *304*, 1191–1197. [CrossRef]
40. Weiner, S.J. Advancing Health Equity by Avoiding Judgmentalism and Contextualizing Care. *AMA J. Ethics* **2021**, *23*, E91–E96. [CrossRef]
41. Dayton, E.; Henriksen, K. Communication failure: Basic components, contributing factors, and the call for structure. *Jt. Comm. J. Qual. Patient Saf.* **2007**, *33*, 34–47. [CrossRef]
42. Haynes, A.B.; Weiser, T.G.; Berry, W.R.; Lipsitz, S.R.; Breizat, A.H.; Dellinger, E.P.; Herbosa, T.; Joseph, S.; Kibatala, P.L.; Lapitan, M.C.; et al. A surgical safety checklist to reduce morbidity and mortality in a global population. *N. Engl. J. Med.* **2009**, *360*, 491–499. [CrossRef]
43. Müller, M.; Jürgens, J.; Redaèlli, M.; Klingberg, K.; Hautz, W.E.; Stock, S. Impact of the communication and patient hand-off tool SBAR on patient safety: A systematic review. *BMJ Open* **2018**, *8*, e022202. [CrossRef]
44. Ruhomauly, Z.; Betts, K.; Jayne-Coupe, K.; Karanfilian, L.; Szekely, M.; Relwani, A.; McCay, J.; Jaffry, Z. Improving the quality of handover: Implementing SBAR. *Future Healthc. J.* **2019**, *6* (Suppl. 2), 54. [CrossRef]
45. Reichman, V.; Brachio, S.S.; Madu, C.R.; Montoya-Williams, D.; Peña, M.M. Using rising tides to lift all boats: Equity-focused quality improvement as a tool to reduce neonatal health disparities. *Semin. Fetal Neonatal Med.* **2021**, *26*, 101198. [CrossRef]
46. Colldén, C.; Hellström, A.; Gremyr, I. Value configurations for balancing standardization and customization in chronic care: A qualitative study. *BMC Health Serv. Res.* **2021**, *21*, 845. [CrossRef] [PubMed]
47. Cooper, A.B.; Chidwick, P.; Cybulski, P.; Sibbald, R. Checklist to meet Ethical and Legal Obligations in the consent pathway for critically ill patients (ChELO): A quality improvement project and case studies. *Can. J. Crit. Care Nurs.* **2015**, *26*, 16–24. [PubMed]

children

MDPI

Article

Human Milk Fatty Acid Composition and Its Effect on Preterm Infants' Growth Velocity

Batool Ahmed [1], Afnan Freije [1], Amina Omran [1], Mariangela Rondanelli [2,3], Mirko Marino [4] and Simone Perna [4,*]

[1] Department of Biology, College of Science, University of Bahrain, Sakhir 32038, Bahrain
[2] IRCCS Mondino Foundation, 27100 Pavia, Italy
[3] Unit of Human and Clinical Nutrition, Department of Public Health, Experimental and Forensic Medicine, University of Pavia, 27100 Pavia, Italy
[4] Department of Food, Environmental and Nutritional Sciences (DeFENS), Division of Human Nutrition, Università degli Studi di Milano, 20133 Milan, Italy; marino@unimi.it
* Correspondence: simone.perna@unimi.it

Abstract: This study aimed to analyze the fatty acid content in human milk and to find its relationship with the growth velocity of preterm infants. Mature milk samples from 15 mothers of preterm infants were collected from three different hospitals, followed by lipid extraction, fatty acid methylation, and finally gas chromatography analysis to determine the fatty acids composition. The average total lipid content was 3.61 ± 1.57 g/100 mL with the following classes of fatty acids: saturated fatty acids 43.54 ± 11.16%, unsaturated fatty acids 52.22 ± 10.89%, in which monounsaturated fatty acids were 36.52 ± 13.90%, and polyunsaturated fatty acids were 15.70 ± 7.10%. Polyunsaturated fatty acid sub-class n-6 was 15.23 ± 8.23% and n-3 was 0.46 ± 0.18%. Oleic acid, palmitic acid, and linoleic acid were the most abundant fatty acids. The n-6/n-3 ratio was 32.83:1. EPA and DHA fatty acids were not detected. As gestational age and birth weight increase, C20:2n6 content increases. The growth velocity increases with the decrement in C16 and increment in C20:2n6. The lipid profile of preterm human milk was found to be low in some essential fatty acids, which may affect the quality of preterm infants' nutrition.

Keywords: human milk; fatty acids; preterm; growth velocity

1. Introduction

Breastfeeding is the most common and perfect way in which newborn infants can receive the needed nutrients that help in achieving healthy growth and development in the early stages of life. It is recommended to exclusively breastfed infants for the first hour after delivery and the first 6 months of their life, and then it is advised to continue breastfeeding for 2 years along with the introduction of food [1].

The major source of energy in breastfed infants is fat, which is present in the form of lipid globules that contribute to 40–55% of the total intake of energy [2]. Triacylglycerol (TAG) is the major lipid form present in human milk comprising 98–99% of total lipids. Each TAG consists of a glycerol molecule that is bonded to three fatty acid chains of different lengths. These fatty acids (FAs) can either be saturated fatty acids (SFA) that are characterized by having no double bond in their hydrocarbon chain, monounsaturated (MUFA) that have a single double bond, or polyunsaturated (PUFA) that have more than one double bond in their chain [3]. There are three possible sources of FA in breast milk, and they can come from the maternal diet or mothers' adipose tissues or can be synthesized in mothers' body tissues [4].

Long-chain polyunsaturated fatty acids (LC-PUFAs), which have ≥18 carbons in the chain, play important roles during the pregnancy of the woman and after the birth for both mother and infant [5]. During pregnancy, LC-PUFAs ensure the proper growth of the fetus and reduce the chances of preterm birth [6], whereas after birth they help in regulating growth, developing the immune system functions, improving the allergic and inflammatory responses, and developing the motor and the nervous system [7,8].

As shown by different references, infants born smaller than average are more likely to face certain diseases during their life [1]. Preterm infants, who are born less than 32 weeks of gestation, require higher amounts of nutrients than term infants due to the immaturity of their gastrointestinal tract and rapid growth rate [9,10]. Mother's milk has proven to be the most suitable feeding strategy for preterm infants [11]. It was found that human milk reduced the incidence of necrotizing enterocolitis (NEC) and sepsis during their hospital stay [12]. Furthermore, it reduced the morbidity and mortality rates at NICUs. In addition, it enhanced the neurodevelopment of these infants [13]. Due to its variability between mothers and within different lactation periods, infants may suffer from a shortage in their nutrition [14]. Dror and Allen (2018) suggested that human milk lipid content may not change with the maternal diet, but fatty acids can be modified [15]. Innis (2004) found that unsaturated FAs are highly affected by the quality of maternal intake of FAs [16]. Little is known about the effect of different FAs on preterm infants' growth, and such knowledge is needed to improve the feeding and fortification strategies used in neonatal intensive care units (NICUs) to achieve the best growth outcomes. This study aims to assess the FA profile of human breast milk from mothers who delivered preterm infants and to assess its effect on preterm infant growth velocity for 30 days of their hospital stay. To our knowledge, this is the first study in the Kingdom of Bahrain that addresses this issue and analyzes human milk for its fatty acids. This will provide baseline data for future research.

2. Materials and Methods

2.1. Study Design

This study is a continuation of the pilot study of Ahmed et al. (2021), which aimed to assess the effect of human milk energy and macronutrient content on preterm infants' growth rate [17]. It was conducted between July 2018 and March 2021 at the NICUs of the three main hospitals in the Kingdom of Bahrain, Salmaniya Medical Complex (SMC), Bahrain Defence Force Royal Medical Services (BDF) and King Hamad University Hospital (KHUH). Fifteen lactating mothers of healthy preterm infants, born with a birth weight less than 1500 g or with a gestational age of less than 32 weeks, and receiving their mother's milk, participated in this study. Basic data of infants, including gestational age (weeks), birth weight (kg), daily weight (kg), and weekly head circumference (cm), were collected from their medical records. Growth velocity (GV) for 30 days or until discharge was calculated in g/kg/day as suggested by Patel et al. (2009) [18], and head circumference growth rate (cm/week) was calculated by taking the average of the readings for 4 weeks or until discharge. All this was started when infants reached full feed of 120 mL/kg/day of expressed breast milk and discontinuation of intravenous infusion. Some infants received fortified expressed breast milk and preterm formula milk as prescribed by their physician for a few days during the study.

2.2. Sample Collection

Milk samples were collected two weeks after delivery by the mothers when the milk composition was more stable (mature milk) [19], either at home or at the hospital using electrical pumps. The samples were collected once a week for only two constitutive weeks. Two samples, 5 mL each, were collected each day (from morning and evening expressions) and pooled in one breast-milk storage bag to exclude diurnal variation in milk composition. Milk samples were stored at −100 °C freezer until analysis. The samples were thawed at 37 °C water bath and vortexed for 30 s before analysis.

2.3. Lipid Extraction and Methylation

Total lipids were first extracted from the milk using the Folch et al. (1957) method [20]. Nineteen ml of (2:1) chloroform–methanol solution was added to 4 mL of the milk sample and vortexed for 10 min, and then 4 mL of deionized water was added, and the tubes were vortexed again for 10 min. To separate the mixture into two phases, centrifugation was performed at 2400 rpm for 20 min. In a pre-weighed tube, the lower phase was transferred and dried under the nitrogen gas in a 37 °C water bath until a clear oil was formed. Total lipids were expressed as g/100 mL of human milk.

This was followed by FA methylation according to the modifications that were conducted by Ozogul et al. (2012) to the Association of Official Analytical Chemists (AOAC) procedures (1990) [21,22]. The whole extracted milk lipid was mixed with 1.5 mL of 0.5 M methanolic sodium hydroxide, and then heated for 7 min at 100 °C and left to cool down at room temperature. After the addition of 2 mL of 14% boron trifluoride-methanol to the mixture, it was heated for 5 min at 100 °C and cooled down to 30–40 °C. One ml of isooctane was added to the tube and vortexed for 30 s. Immediately, 5 mL of saturated sodium chloride was added, and shaking was applied for 30 s. The tube was left to allow the separation of the layers. The isooctane upper layer was placed in another tube and 1 mL of isooctane was added to the mixture again and vortexed for 30 s, and it was left to separate, and the upper layer was removed. After combining the two isooctane extract layers, they were dried under nitrogen gas to 1 mL.

2.4. Gas Chromatography

A Perkin Elmer, Clarus 500 GC-FID gas chromatography (GC) equipped with Flame Ionization Detector (FID) and Thermal Conductivity Detector (TCD) was used for the analysis of fatty acids. Using a 30 m × 0.25 mm × 0.25 µm fused carbon-silica column with a temperature range from 40 °C to 260 °C (Stabilwax, Crossbond, Carbowax, Polyethylene glycol), the individual fatty acid methyl esters (FAMEs) were separated. The temperatures were set at 200 °C for the GC oven, 300 °C for FID, 150 °C for TCD, and 250 °C for the injector with a split ratio of 1:2. The flow rate for the carrier gas (nitrogen) was 0.76 mL/min and for the other gases was 450 mL/min for air and 45 mL/min for hydrogen. The injection volume of the sample was 5 µL and the sampling rate was 12.5 Hz. Eighty minutes was set as the total run time for each sample. PUFA No.1 (Marine source) and PUFA No.2 (Animal source) supplied by SUPELCO (USA) were used as an authentic FAMEs standard for identification according to the retention time. FAs to be detected were like the PUFAs used, which ranged from C14 to C24. Values of FAs were expressed as mg/100 mL of human milk and g/100 g of FAs (%).

2.5. Statistical Analysis

The data were processed in Microsoft Excel 2010 (Microsoft Corp., Redmond, WA, USA). The normal distribution of the variables was checked using the Shapiro-Wilks test and using Q-Q graphs.

Results of basic characteristics and FA classes were reported as mean ± standard deviation (SD), while FA profiles were reported as mean, variance, SD, minimum (Min), and maximum (Max) in mg/100 mL of human milk and % of fatty acids. Jeffrey's Amazing Statistics Program (JASP) (JASP Team (2022). JASP (Version 0.16.2) [Computer software]) was used to find the effect of gestational age, birth weight, and GV, on the FA composition of human milk using Kendall's tau-b correlation coefficient (r). Scattered plots were used to demonstrate the significant correlations. p-values of <0.05 were set as significance level.

3. Results

3.1. Descriptive Data

The basic characteristics of 19 preterm infants of the participated mothers and the mean total lipid content of collected milk samples are described in Table 1. Most of the infants were males (n = 11) and twins (n = 11). Fourteen of them were delivered by cesarean section and the rest were delivered by normal or spontaneous vaginal delivery. The GV for only 4 preterm infants was calculated for 15 days instead of 30 days due to discharge. All infants received expressed own mother's milk every day during the study. Nine infants did not receive any fortified milk or formula milk. The average number of days infants received fortified milk was 6.3 days, while the average number of days infants received formula milk was 8.6 days. More demographic and anthropometric data of the recruited preterm infants are present in the study of Ahmed et al. (2021) [17].

Table 1. Preterm infant's basic characteristics.

Characteristic	Mean ± SD
Gestational age at birth (weeks)	28.09 ± 2.33
Birth weight (kg)	1.14 ± 0.353
Growth velocity (GV) (g/kg/day)	13.85 ± 4.10
Head circumference growth rate (HC) (cm/week)	0.63 ± 0.18
Total lipids (g/100 mL)	3.61 ± 1.57

SD: Standard deviation.

3.2. Classes of Fatty Acids in Human Milk

Table 2 summarizes the sum of SFAs, unsaturated fatty acids (UFAs), MUFAs, PUFAs, omega-6 (ω-6, n-6), and omega-3 (ω-3, n-3) that were found in human milk in two units (mg/100 mL) and (%).

Table 2. The sum of different classes of fatty acids in human milk.

Fatty Acids Classes	Mean ± SD mg/100 mL	Mean ± SD %
Σ SFAs	852.10 ± 234.80	43.54 ± 11.16
Σ UFAs	1079.02 ± 227.05	52.22 ±10.89
Σ MUFAs	761.02 ± 291.28	36.52 ± 13.90
Σ PUFAs	318.00 ± 142.92	15.70 ± 7.10
Σ n-6	307.98 ± 165.59	15.23 ±8.23
Σ n-3	10.02 ± 6.84	0.46 ± 0.18
n-6/n-3 ratio	30.73:1	32.83:1

MUFAs: Monounsaturated fatty acids, n-3: Omega-3, n-6: Omega-6, PUFAs: Polyunsaturated fatty acids, SD: Standard deviation, SFAs: Saturated fatty acids, UFAs: Unsaturated fatty acids.

The data show that the UFA class is greater than the SFAs, accounting for more than half the total lipids. In the UFAs, the MUFAs were the highest, accounting for 69.94% of the UFAs, followed were the PUFAs with 30.07% of UFAs. The PUFAs were found to be mostly n-6 FAs (97.01% of PUFAs), while n-3 represented only 2.99% of the PUFAs.

3.3. Fatty Acid Profile of Human Milk Samples

Thirteen FAs were found in approximately all milk samples. In the SFAs, (C14:0, C16:0, C20:0, and C18:0) were seen. It was found that the palmitic acid (C16:0) comprised the highest value and (C18:3n6) was the lowest one. In the MUFAs, five FAs were found: (C16:1n9, C16:1n7, C18:1n9, C18:1n7, and C20:1n9), with oleic acid (C18:1n9) being the highest and palmitoleic acid (C16:1n7) being the lowest. In the PUFAs, four FAs were found: (C18:2n6, C18:3n-6, C18:3n-3, and C20:2n6) with linoleic acid (C18:2n6) being the highest value and γ-linolenic acid (C18:3n6) being the lowest. Three n-6 FAs were detected, (C18:2n6, C18:3n-6, and C20:2n6), with the linoleic acid (C18:2n6) being the highest one and γ-linolenic acid (C18:3n6) being the lowest one. Only one n-3 FA was detected, while α-linolenic acid (C18:3n3), Eicosapentaenoic acid (EPA) and Docosahexaenoic acid (DHA) were not detected. The absolute values (mg/100 mL) were converted to relative values (%), where oleic acid (C18:1n9) was the highest and γ-linolenic acid (C18:3n6) was the lowest (Table 3).

Table 3. The fatty acid profile in the milk samples of the preterm infant that was collected postpartum expressed as (mg/100 mL) of milk and % of fatty acids.

Fatty Acids	mg/100 mL of Human Milk					% of Fatty Acids				
	Mean	Var	SD	Min	Max	Mean	Var	SD	Min	Max
14:0	211.60	6848.97	82.76	61.96	335.51	11.67	17.70	4.21	6.03	19.01
16:0	526.41	54,281.49	232.98	114.12	955.30	26.12	11.37	3.37	19.82	31.47
16:1n9	50.83	769.71	27.74	10.31	103.08	2.51	0.55	0.74	0.57	3.41
16:1n7	6.04	111.35	10.55	0.78	44.97	0.27	0.18	0.42	0.09	1.85
18:0	107.91	2380.59	48.79	27.36	179.40	5.43	0.79	0.89	3.93	7.06
18:1n9	672.33	113,088.66	336.29	103.54	1301.31	32.12	16.62	4.08	26.04	41.30
18:1n7	21.45	221.37	14.88	6.43	66.54	1.13	0.24	0.49	0.38	1.93
18:2n6	293.85	20,688.57	143.84	42.66	550.22	14.58	10.38	3.22	11.01	21.42
18:3n6	5.17	22.55	4.75	0.00	20.35	0.22	0.03	0.18	0.00	0.84
18:3n3	10.02	46.82	6.84	1.32	28.36	0.46	0.03	0.18	0.27	0.90
20:0	6.18	10.68	3.27	1.63	13.45	0.33	0.01	0.11	0.18	0.61
20:1n9	10.37	29.50	5.43	0.00	22.36	0.50	0.04	0.20	0.00	0.82
20:2n6	8.96	22.40	4.73	0.00	18.96	0.43	0.03	0.18	0.00	0.73

Max: Maximum value, Min: Minimum value, SD: Standard deviation, Var: Variance, Mean: mean of cases.

Figure 1 represents the significant correlations found between birth weight, gestational age at birth, and growth velocity of preterm infants and the FA content of the milk samples. Positive correlations were found between birth weight and gestational age with eicosadienoic acid (C20:2n6) ($r = 0.404$, $p = 0.017$; $r = 0.563$, $p = 0.001$), respectively. A strong negative correlation was found between growth velocity and C16:0 FA ($r = -0.538$, $p = 0.001$), but positively correlated to C20:2n6 ($r = 0.491$, $p = 0.004$). No other significant correlations were found between birth weight, gestational age at birth, and GV with the rest of the FAs.

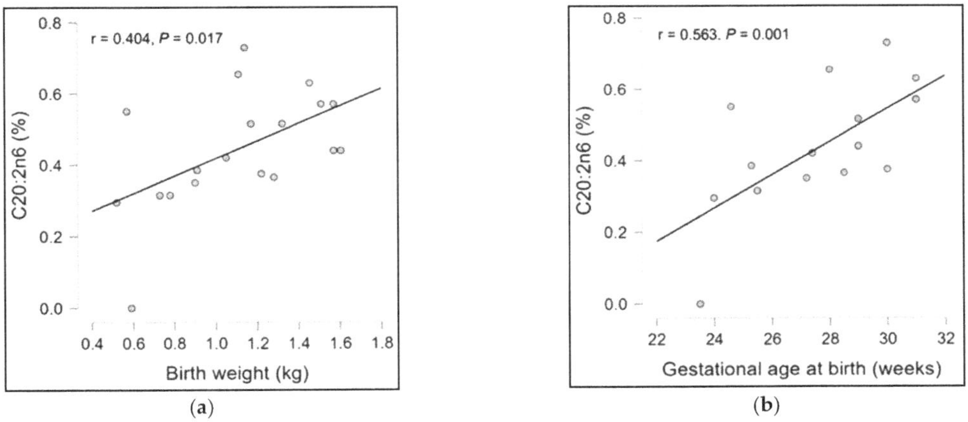

Figure 1. *Cont.*

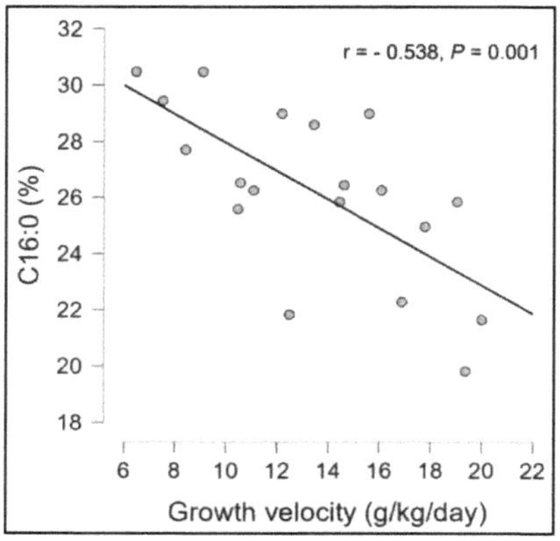

(**c**)

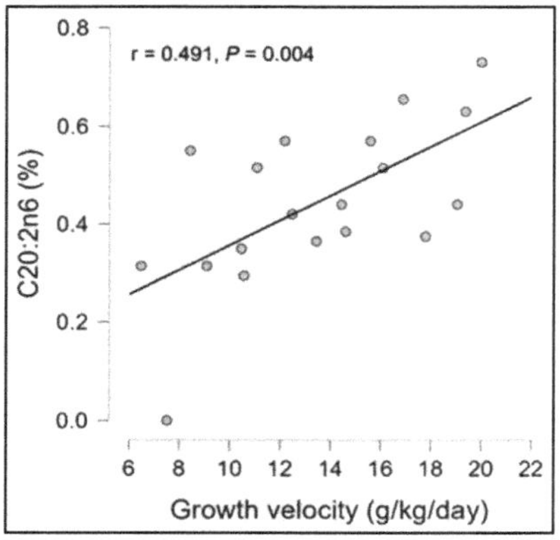

(**d**)

Figure 1. The effect of (**a**) birth weight, (**b**) gestational age at birth, and (**c**,**d**) growth velocity on the fatty acid content of mother's milk in g/100 g (%) of total fatty acids.

4. Discussion

The lipid profile of preterm human milk was found to be low in some essential FAs, which may affect the quality of preterm infants' nutrition.

The SFAs detected in this study were the medium-chain FAs (C14:0), long-chain FAs (C16:0, C18:0), and very long-chain FAs (C20:0). In the present study, the sum of SFAs (43.54 ± 11.16%) was close to the study conducted by Thakkar et al. (2019) (45.88 ± 7.45%) [23]. By contrast, Wan et al. (2010) and Miliku et al. (2019) found a lower value (35.92 ± 7.34%, 39.75 ± 5.00%, respectively) [24,25].

Palmitic acid (C16:0) was the dominant SFA in the present study (26.12 ± 3.37%), which was consistent with the above studies. A negative correlation was found between palmitic acid (C16:0) and growth velocity. Palmitic acid can be endogenously synthesized from glucose in the liver [26]; because the gestational age increases, the development of the body organs will be fully completed and they will function accurately, and hence the functional requirement for the palmitic acid will be decreased. It was found that 10–12% of the total energy intake comes from palmitic acid [27]. The study by Ahmed et al. (2021) found that preterm infants that were fed human milk with less total lipids than the recommended amount (4.4–6.0 g/100 kcal) had better weight gain rates, most probably due to the reduced protein oxidation by lipids as a result of using carbohydrates as an energy source instead of lipids [17,28].

The MUFAs accounted for (36.52 ± 13.90%) of the total FA content, which was slightly higher than the study conducted by Wan et al. (2010) with a value of 32.59% (±7.21%) [24]. However, it was lower than the studies by Miliku et al. (2019) and Thakkar et al. (2019) with the values of 43.06% (±3.59%) and 40.44% (±5.6%) [23,25]. Overall, the MUFAs were the most abundant FAs in the UFA class in all these studies including the present study. Oleic acid (C18:1n9) was found to be the most abundant MUFA (32.12 ± 4.08%), which was similar to the studies by Wan et al. (2010) (31.26 ± 3.72%), Miliku et al. (2019) (37.05 ± 3.59%), and Thakkar et al. (2019) (35.22 ± 5.16%), comprising 88% of the total MUFAs [23–25]. The PUFAs comprised 15.70% (±7.10%) of the total FAs, which is similar to the value found by Koletzko (2016) (15.2 ± 4.26 %) Bzikowska-Jura et al. (2019) (15.1 ± 3.4%) and Freitas et al. (2020) (14.94 ± 5.07%) [29–31]. A positive relationship was found between the gestational age (r = 0.563, $p < 0.001$), birth weight (r = 0.404, $p < 0.017$), and growth velocity (r = 0.491, $p < 0.004$) with Eicosadienoic acid (C20:2n6 %). It was found that n-6 LC-PUFA had a protective effect against intestinal injury in the murine model, reducing inflammation and intestinal damage by increasing the lipoxin A4 levels [32]. This may explain the need for this FA for preterm infants who have immature intestines and help to reduce the incidence of NEC.

Only one n-3 FA, namely α-linolenic acid (C18:3n3), was found in the current study; this finding was not in agreement with other studies where they found more than one n-3, including EPA (C20:5n3) and DHA(C22:6n3) [25,29]. Very few studies could not detect the EPA and DHA; one of them is the study conducted in Brazil by Freitas et al. (2020) where the only n-3 FA found was α-linolenic acid (C18:3n3), which is consistent with this study [31].

A study conducted by Bzikowska-Jura et al. (2019) investigated the association between the n-3 FA levels and their maternal current dietary intake and habitual dietary intake. They found that the frequency of food products and fish intake had a positive correlation with the concentrations of α-linolenic acid, EPA, and DHA in human milk [30].

Miliku et al. (2019) found that milk samples from mothers who were not taking fish oil supplements had the lowest EPA and DHA levels (0.07% and 0.16%) in comparison to mothers who were taking them during pregnancy (0.10% and 0.23%) and lactation (0.13% and 0.27%). Their study also showed that the fish oil supplements had a positive association with the high n-3 pattern and negative associations with the high n-6 pattern and n-6/n-3 ratio, where the ratio changed from 6.63% with no supplementation to 6.14% with supplementation ($p < 0.01$), and similar results were found for the intake of shellfish, white fish and fatty cold-water fish [25].

A study conducted in the Kingdom of Bahrain by Freije (2009) showed that the EPA and DHA levels in local fish ranged from 0.030 to 0.239 g/3oz, which was much lower than the range recommended by the USDA Nutrient Data Laboratory (0.13–1.81 g/3oz), and this accounts for the low EPA and DHA intake (0.02–0.13 g/day) that does not meet the recommended value (0.3–0.5 g/day) [29]. Accordingly, the absence of EPA and DHA in the present study can be attributed to the low maternal intake frequency of foods high in n-3 (fish and seafood), the low n-3 quality in the local fish, as well as not taking n-3 supplements during pregnancy and the lactation period [25,30,33].

The GV of the study sample was found to be less than the recommended values (GV = 15–20 g/kg/day) [34]. Much et al. (2013) found that 3-n LCPUFA is responsible for increasing fat mass over the first year of a newborn's life. Unfortunately, it was possible to compare 3-n LCPUFA because EPA and DHA were missing. However, this can also explain the low GV of the study subjects [35].

In the present study, the n-6/n-3 ratio was 32.83:1, which was much higher than the other studies, such as those by Thakkar et al. (2019) (9.72 ± 4.94%) and Miliku et al. (2019) (6.53 ± 1.72%), and this was due to the very low sum of n-3 fatty acids (0.46 ± 0.18%) found in this study in comparison to the previous studies by Thakkar et al. (2019) (1.15 ± 0.62%), Wan et al. (2010) (1.22 ± 0.29%), and Miliku et al. (2019) (2.39 ± 0.7%) [23–25].. The high n-6 in the Westernized diet can be due to the evolution of modern agriculture, agribusiness, processed food, and the production of hydrogenated and refined vegetable oil [36–40].

It is important to inspect the role of eicosadienoic acid (C20:2n6) in preterm growth and quantify the best amount needed to obtain the best growth outcome for infants. This information can be used for the improvement of a lactating mother's diet or the introduction of n-3 supplements to reduce the n-6/n-3 ratio. In addition, it can be used in the manufacturing of milk fortifiers and preterm infants' formula milk. Additionally, the infants included in this study did not receive any antibiotics or probiotics during the observation.

The main limitation of the study is the low sample size of the subjects due to the low number of eligible mothers and preterm infants for the study criteria and the low participation rate. A study with a larger sample size is recommended to be conducted before the implementation of the recommendations. The essential FAs such as EPA and DHA were missing, which prevents the human milk from being sufficient for providing the optimum nutrition required for the growth and development of the preterm infant.

Another limitation is that it was difficult to compare results with other studies that use different units of measurement (ounces instead of grams).

5. Conclusions

To our knowledge, this is the first study conducted in the Kingdom of Bahrain to evaluate human milk. The lipid profile of preterm human milk was found to be low in some essential FAs, which may affect the quality of preterm infants' nutrition. Eicosadienoic acid (C20:2n6) was found to positively affect the growth velocity of preterm infants, which may be due to reducing inflammation and intestinal injury. Another key finding was that a negative correlation was found between palmitic acid (C16:0) and growth velocity which could be due to reduced protein oxidation by lipids. Unfortunately, EPA and DHA were not detected, which indicates that preterm infants may receive milk poor in n-3 FA. Mothers need to increase their n-3 FA intake either by food or supplements to eliminate its deficiency. Further investigation with a larger sample size is needed to confirm the study's findings.

Author Contributions: Conceptualization, B.A., S.P. and A.F.; methodology, A.F.; software, S.P.; validation, A.F.; formal analysis, S.P.; investigation, B.A. and A.O.; resources, A.F.; data curation, B.A., M.M.; writing—original draft preparation, A.O., S.P. and B.A.; writing—review and editing, B.A., M.R., M.M. and A.F.; visualization, B.A., M.M.; supervision, A.F.; project administration, A.F. All authors have read and agreed to the published version of the manuscript.

Funding: This research received no external funding.

Institutional Review Board Statement: The study was conducted in accordance with the Declaration of Helsinki, and approved by the Institutional Review Board (or Ethics Committee) of Ministry of Health Technical Support Team (RTST) Committee (AUHR/457/2018) 1/05/2018 and the three main hospitals in the Kingdom of Bahrain, Salmaniya Medical Complex (SMC) Secondary Health Care Research Sub-Committee (SHCRC), Bahrain Defence Force Royal Medical Services (BDF) Research Ethics Committee (BDF/R&REC/2019-331), and King Hamad University Hospital (KHUH) Research and Ethics Committee (Ref.KHUH/Research/No.286/2019).

Informed Consent Statement: Informed consent was obtained from all subjects involved in the study.

Data Availability Statement: Not applicable.

Acknowledgments: The authors acknowledge the support of the APC central fund of the University of Milano. The authors acknowledge Fatima Alhakim and Ahmed Elbehery, who collected milk samples and infants' data.

Conflicts of Interest: The authors declare no conflict of interest.

References

1. American Academy of Pediatrics. Policy statement: Breastfeeding and the use of human milk. *Pediatrics* **2012**, *129*, e827–e841. [CrossRef] [PubMed]
2. Koletzko, B.; Rodriguez-Palmero, M.; Demmelmair, H.; Fidler, N.; Jensen, R.; Sauerwald, T. Physiological aspects of human milk lipids. *Early Hum. Dev.* **2001**, *65*, S3–S18. [CrossRef] [PubMed]
3. Mazzocchi, A.; D'Oria, V.; Cosmi, V.D.; Bettocchi, S.; Milani, G.P.; Silano, M.; Agostoni, C. The role of lipids in human milk and infant formulae. *Nutrients* **2018**, *10*, 567. [CrossRef] [PubMed]
4. Innis, S.M. Human milk: Maternal dietary lipids and infant development. *Proc. Nutr. Soc.* **2007**, *66*, 397–404. [CrossRef] [PubMed]
5. Kilari, A.S.; Mehendale, S.S.; Dangat, K.D.; Yadav, H.R.; Gupta, A.; Taralekar, V.S.; Joshi, S.R. Long chain polyunsaturated fatty acids in mothers of preterm babies. *J. Perinat. Med.* **2010**, *38*, 659–664. [CrossRef]
6. Duttaroy, A.K.; Basak, S. Maternal dietary fatty acids and their roles in human placental development. *Prostaglandins Leukot. Essent. Fatty Acids* **2020**, *155*, 102080. [CrossRef]
7. Van Elten, T.M.; van Rossem, L.; Wijga, A.H.; Brunekreef, B.; De Jongste, J.C.; Koppelman, G.H.; Smit, H.A. Breast milk fatty acid composition has a long-term effect on the risk of asthma, eczema, and sensitization. *Allergy* **2015**, *70*, 1468–1476. [CrossRef]
8. Hurtado, J.A.; Iznaola, C.; Peña, M.; Ruíz, J.; Peña-Quintana, L.; Kajarabille, N.; Rodriguez-Santana, Y.; Sanjurjo, P.; Aldámiz-Echevarría, L.; Ochoa, J.; et al. Effects of maternal Ω-3 supplementation on fatty acids and on visual and cognitive development. *J. Pediatr. Gastroenterol. Nutr.* **2015**, *61*, 472–480. [CrossRef]

9. Schanler, R.J.; Hurst, N.M.; Lau, C. The use of human milk and breastfeeding in premature infants. *Clin. Perinatol.* **1999**, *26*, 379–398. [CrossRef]
10. Callen, J.; Pinelli, J. A review of the literature examining the benefits and challenges, incidence and duration, and barriers to breastfeeding in preterm infants. *Adv. Neonatal. Care* **2005**, *5*, 72–88. [CrossRef]
11. Ziegler, E.E. Human milk and human milk fortifiers. *Nutr. Care Preterm Infants* **2014**, *110*, 215–227. [CrossRef]
12. Ehrenkranz, R.A.; Dusick, A.M.; Vohr, B.R.; Wright, L.L.; Wrage, L.A.; Poole, W.K.; National Institutes of Child Health and Human Development Neonatal Research Network. Growth in the neonatal intensive care unit influences neurodevelopmental and growth outcomes of extremely low birth weight infants. *Pediatrics* **2006**, *117*, 1253–1261. [CrossRef] [PubMed]
13. Quigley, M.; Embleton, N.D.; McGuire, W. Formula versus donor breast milk for feeding preterm or low birth weight infants. *Cochrane Database Syst. Rev.* **2018**, *6*, CD002971. [CrossRef]
14. Moltó-Puigmartí, C.; Castellote, A.I.; Carbonell-Estrany, X.; López-Sabater, M.C. Differences in fat content and fatty acid proportions among colostrum, transitional, and mature milk from women delivering very preterm, preterm, and term infants. *Clin. Nutr.* **2011**, *30*, 116–123. [CrossRef] [PubMed]
15. Dror, D.K.; Allen, L.H. Overview of nutrients in human milk. *Adv. Nutr.* **2018**, *9* (Suppl. S1), 278S–294S. [CrossRef] [PubMed]
16. Innis, S.M. Polyunsaturated fatty acids in human milk: An essential role in infant development. *Adv. Exp. Med. Biol.* **2004**, *554*, 27–43. [PubMed]
17. Ahmed, B.; Freije, A.; Alhakim, F.; Alhaddad, F.; Elbehery, A.; Perna, S. The Effects of Energy and Macronutrient Content of Human Milk on the Growth of Preterm Infants: A Prospective Cohort Pilot Study. *Bahrain Med. Bull.* **2021**, *43*, 560–566.
18. Patel, A.L.; Engstrom, J.L.; Meier, P.P.; Jegier, B.J.; Kimura, R.E. Calculating postnatal growth velocity in very low birth weight (VLBW) premature infants. *J. Perinatol.* **2009**, *29*, 618–622. [CrossRef]
19. Ballard, O.; Morrow, A.L. Human milk composition: Nutrients and bioactive factors. *Pediatr. Clin. N. Am.* **2013**, *60*, 49–74. [CrossRef]
20. Folch, J.; Lees, M.; Stanley, G.S. A simple method for the isolation and purification of total lipides from animal tissues. *J. Biol. Chem.* **1957**, *226*, 497–509. [CrossRef]
21. Ozogul, Y.; Şimşek, A.; BalIkçI, E.; Kenar, M. The effects of extraction methods on the contents of fatty acids, especially EPA and DHA in marine lipids. *Int. J. Food Sci. Nutr.* **2012**, *63*, 326–331. [CrossRef] [PubMed]
22. Association of Official Analytical Chemists. *Official Methods of Analysis: Changes in Official Methods of Analysis Made at the Annual Meeting*; Association of Official Analytical Chemists: Rockville, ML, USA, 1990.
23. Thakkar, S.K.; De Castro, C.A.; Beauport, L.; Tolsa, J.F.; Fischer Fumeaux, C.J.; Affolter, M.; Giuffrida, F. Temporal progression of fatty acids in preterm and term human milk of mothers from Switzerland. *Nutrients* **2019**, *11*, 112. [CrossRef] [PubMed]
24. Wan, Z.X.; Wang, X.L.; Xu, L.; Geng, Q.; Zhang, Y. Lipid content and fatty acids composition of mature human milk in rural North China. *Br. J. Nutr.* **2010**, *103*, 913–916. [CrossRef]
25. Miliku, K.; Duan, Q.L.; Moraes, T.J.; Becker, A.B.; Mandhane, P.J.; Turvey, S.E.; Lefebvre, D.L.; Sears, M.R.; Subbarao, P.; Field, C.J.; et al. Human milk fatty acid composition is associated with dietary, genetic, sociodemographic, and environmental factors in the CHILD Cohort Study. *Am. J. Clin. Nutr.* **2019**, *110*, 1370–1383. [CrossRef] [PubMed]
26. Donnelly, K.L.; Smith, C.I.; Schwarzenberg, S.J.; Jessurun, J.; Boldt, M.D.; Parks, E.J. Sources of fatty acids stored in liver and secreted via lipoproteins in patients with nonalcoholic fatty liver disease. *J. Clin. Investig.* **2005**, *115*, 1343–1351. [CrossRef]
27. Innis, S.M. Dietary triacylglycerol structure and its role in infant nutrition. *Adv. Nutr.* **2011**, *2*, 275–283. [CrossRef]
28. Kashyap, S.; Towers, H.M.; Sahni, R.; Ohira-Kist, K.; Abildskov, K.; Schulze, K.F. Effects of quality of energy on substrate oxidation in enterally fed, low-birth-weight infants. *Am. J. Clin. Nutr.* **2001**, *74*, 374–380. [CrossRef]
29. Koletzko, B. Human milk lipids. *Ann. Nutr. Metab.* **2016**, *69* (Suppl. S2), 27–40. [CrossRef]
30. Bzikowska-Jura, A.; Czerwonogrodzka-Senczyna, A.; Jasińska-Melon, E.; Mojska, H.; Olędzka, G.; Wesołowska, A.; Szostak-Węgierek, D. The concentration of omega-3 fatty acids in human milk is related to their habitual but not current intake. *Nutrients* **2019**, *11*, 1585. [CrossRef]
31. Freitas, R.F.; Macedo, M.D.; Lessa, A.D.; Ferraz, V.P.; Soares, N.O.; Martins, B.E.; Pinto, N.A.; Teixeira, R.A. Composition in fatty acids of mature milk of nursing mothers. *Rev. Bras. Saúde Matern. Infant.* **2020**, *19*, 817–825. [CrossRef]
32. Gobbetti, T.; Ducheix, S.; Le Faouder, P.; Perez, T.; Riols, F.; Boué, J.; Bertrand-Michel, J.; Dubourdeau, M.; Guillou, H.; Perretti, M.; et al. Protective effects of n-6 fatty acids-enriched diet on intestinal ischaemia/reperfusion injury involve lipoxin A 4 and its receptor. *Br. J. Pharmacol.* **2015**, *172*, 910–923. [CrossRef] [PubMed]
33. Freije, A. Fatty acid profile of the erythrocyte membranes of healthy Bahraini citizens in comparison with coronary heart disease patients. *J. Oleo Sci.* **2009**, *58*, 379–388. [CrossRef] [PubMed]
34. Ehrenkranz, R.A.; Younes, N.; Lemons, J.A.; Fanaroff, A.A.; Donovan, E.F.; Wright, L.L.; Katsikiotis, V.; Tyson, J.E.; Oh, W.; Shankaran, S.; et al. Longitudinal growth of hospitalized very low birth weight infants. *Pediatrics* **1999**, *104*, 280–289. [CrossRef] [PubMed]
35. Much, D.; Brunner, S.; Vollhardt, C.; Schmid, D.; Sedlmeier, E.-M.; Brüderl, M.; Heimberg, E.; Bartke, N.; Boehm, G.; Bader, B.L.; et al. Breast milk fatty acid profile in relation to infant growth and body composition: Results from the INFAT study. *Pediatr. Res.* **2013**, *74*, 230–237. [CrossRef] [PubMed]
36. Simopoulos, A.P. Importance of the omega-6/omega-3 balance in health and disease: Evolutionary aspects of diet. In *Healthy Agriculture, Healthy Nutrition, Healthy People*; Karger Publishers: Basel, Switzerland, 2011; Volume 102, pp. 10–21.

37. Simopoulos, A.P. An increase in the omega-6/omega-3 fatty acid ratio increases the risk for obesity. *Nutrients* **2016**, *8*, 128. [CrossRef]
38. Chaves, H.; Singh, R.B.; Khan, S.; Wilczynska, A.; Takahashi, T. High omega-6/omega-3 fatty acid ratio diets and risk of noncommunicable diseases: Is the tissue, the main issue? In *The Role of Functional Food Security in Global Health*; Academic Press: Cambridge, MA, USA, 2019; pp. 217–259. [CrossRef]
39. Saini, R.K.; Keum, Y.S. Omega-3 and omega-6 polyunsaturated fatty acids: Dietary sources, metabolism, and significance—A review. *Life Sci.* **2018**, *203*, 255–267. [CrossRef]
40. Bhardwaj, K.; Verma, N.; Trivedi, R.K.; Bhardwaj, S.; Shukla, N. Significance of ratio of omega-3 and omega-6 in human health with special reference to flaxseed oil. *Int. J. Biol. Chem.* **2016**, *10*, 1–6. [CrossRef]

children

MDPI

Article

Prenatal Predictors of Neurobehavioral Outcome in Children with Fetal Growth Restriction at 6 Years of Age: A Retrospective Cohort Study

Mª José Benítez Marín [1,2,3,*], Marta Blasco Alonso [2,3,4] and Ernesto González Mesa [2,3,4]

1 Obstetrics and Gynecology Service, Virgen de la Victoria University Hospital, 29010 Málaga, Spain
2 Surgical Specialties, Biochemistry and Immunology Department, Málaga University, 29071 Málaga, Spain; martablascoalonso@gmail.com (M.B.A.); egonzalezmesa@uma.es (E.G.M.)
3 Research Group in Maternal-Fetal Medicine, Epigenetics, Women's Diseases and Reproductive Health, Instituto de Investigación Biomédica de Málaga y Plataforma en Nanomedicina-IBIMA Plataforma Bionand, 29071 Málaga, Spain
4 Obstetrics and Gynecology Service, Regional University Hospital of Malaga, 29011 Málaga, Spain
* Correspondence: mariajosebenitezmarin@gmail.com

Abstract: (1) Background: Fetal growth restriction (FGR) increases the risk of adverse neurodevelopmental outcomes, especially in preterm newborns. This study aims to describe the behavioral results of FGR at 6 years of age and to demonstrate the relationship of certain predictive factors with this development. (2) Methods: This retrospective cohort study included 70 children born in 2015 at the University Hospital Carlos Haya, Málaga, Spain who had been exposed to FGR during pregnancy; neonatal and infant data were recorded retrospectively. Children were assessed prospectively at 6 years of age by means of a strengths and difficulties questionnaire (SDQ) to study behavioral outcomes. (3) Results: We demonstrated that there are higher behavioral disability rates in children exposed to FGR during pregnancy and, in particular, high rates of hyperactivity or conduct problems. We also proved a negative relationship between the birth weight percentile and the total behavioral scale score, along with a positive correlation between hyperactivity and the emotional and behavioral scales. Learning difficulties were more frequent in early-onset FGR than in late-onset FGR. (4) Conclusions: Our study of behavioral development has demonstrated higher behavioral disability rates in children with FGR at 6 years of age; specifically, high rates of hyperactivity or conduct problems. At the same time, we have proved a negative relationship between the birth weight percentile and the total behavioral scale score.

Keywords: fetal growth restriction; neurodevelopment; behavioral; outcomes; cognitive; brain sparing effect

1. Introduction

Fetal growth restriction (FGR) has varied greatly in terms of its management over time. Nowadays, FGR management techniques have improved the standard treatment guidelines. As a result, restriction severity and prematurity issues now have established follow-up and completion dates to reduce perinatal morbidity and mortality [1–3]. Thanks to improvements in pregnancy management, perinatal care, and neonatal techniques, perinatal mortality has decreased considerably, especially in extremely premature infants. However, these improvements may not appreciably reduce perinatal morbidity [4].

Neonatal outcomes in FGR have been exhaustively researched, and prematurity has been strongly associated with short-term outcomes [2]. Childhood development may also be influenced by FGR [5] and interest in long-term outcomes, specifically regarding neurodevelopment, is growing. A considerable number of studies in human and animal models have demonstrated changes to the nervous system's structure, affecting brain volume [6–8], grey matter volume and structure [8–10], and white matter structure and myelinization [11,12], as well as influencing the gyrification process [13] in FGR conditions. These changes may affect motor, cognitive, adaptive, and behavioral development.

However, the results of these studies are often heterogeneous and contradictory. In most cases, assessments may be carried out at very early stages before the development of a given research object's cognitive deficits or behavioral changes. The studies also include a heterogeneous group of children, both those who are small for their gestational age and those with FGR; in many cases, the authors did not take into account the issue of prematurity, which could alter the results. Despite these heterogeneities and contradictions, outcomes such as poor results in intelligence coefficients, poor academic results, cognitive and emotional alterations, and attention and hyperactivity disorders, as well as behavioral disabilities have been described with early-onset FGR. The most severe cases have been linked with motor disorders and cerebral palsy [6,14–20]. These results do not shed much light on late-onset FGR when reaching the gestational term [21–27].

Similarly, various research groups have attempted to show the relationship between different prenatal markers and motor, cognitive, and behavioral development. In our previous systematic review, we were able to associate brain sparing with poorer cognitive development. However, the link between brain sparing effect and behavioral skills development was difficult to establish [28].

In our previous research, we assessed FGR children by means of the Battelle Developmental Inventory (BDI), evaluating milestones in different areas. We found a high rate of poor global development, with motor and communication skills being the main areas affected. Conversely, we were able to associate the brain-sparing effect with worse coefficients of global development. However, the cognitive delay rate was low [29].

It has been shown that early attention and early stimulation in children that are born preterm can have a positive effect on motor neurodevelopment, and that this positive effect on cognition continues into school age [30]. Therefore, the early detection of FGR in neurocognitive risk could allow for the implementation of early stimulation strategies to improve their deficits for a longer period. In the same way, cognitive development and emotional intelligence could be improved, and better resilience and future personal relationships obtained, by identifying and improving the influencing factors (both positive and negative).

We believe that children who have been exposed to FGR during pregnancy have a higher risk of behavioral disorders. This study aims to describe the behavioral results of FGR in children at 6 years of age. Secondly, we demonstrate the relationship of certain predictive factors with this developmental issue, which might help us to select a population that is at risk of FGR, in order to assist with early childhood support or with psychological assessment and management.

2. Methods

2.1. Population

This cohort study had a retrospective design, in which we selected a group of FGR children born in 2015 at University Hospital Carlos Haya, Málaga, Spain. This hospital is a specialized center for the diagnosis and treatment of this pathology. Table 1 describes our inclusion and exclusion criteria, based on the definition of FGR. We define the brain-sparing effect as a cerebroplacental ratio (CPR) below the 5th percentile. When FGR is diagnosed at or below 32 weeks of gestational age, it is defined as early-onset FGR. In the event that this diagnosis is beyond 32 weeks, it is defined as late-onset FGR. Recruitment started in 2021, following approval from the regional ethics committee, and parental consent was obtained before child assessment began. Medical and sociodemographic data were collected from clinical records and parents' reports. This study protocol was previously described in our most recent publication [29].

Table 1. Inclusion and exclusion criteria.

Inclusion Criteria	Exclusion Criteria
Birth weight less than the 3rd percentile	Structural and chromosomal abnormalities Multiple pregnancies Small for gestational age
Birth weight less than the 10th percentile and abnormal Doppler study: - UA-PI above the 95th percentile - MCA-PI below the 5th percentile - CPR below the 5th percentile, or - Uterine arteries-PI above the 95th percentile	
CPR = MCA-PI/UA-PI	

UA-PI: umbilical artery pulsatility index, MCA-PI: middle cerebral artery pulsatility index, CPR: cerebroplacental ratio, PI: pulsatility index.

2.2. Parents' Reports and Data Collection

We examined the pregnancy and neonatal care information given in the medical records and recorded all the variables related to pregnancy care, FGR characteristics, Doppler measurements, and delivery episodes. After birth, we recorded the variables related to neonatal anthropometric measurements, adverse neonatal outcomes, and, if applicable, admission days in the neonatal intensive care unit (NICU).

Parents completed a survey to provide information on sociodemographic items and childhood problems, such as academic difficulties, the need for early child support, kindergarten attendance, or any major health problems.

2.3. Behavioral Assessment

The Spanish version of the strengths and difficulties questionnaire (SDQ) was completed prospectively when the subjects were 6 years of age [31]. This questionnaire provides a brief emotional and behavioral screening test for children that is completed by their parents. It can be used in both low- and high-risk populations [32]. This test consists of 25 items, divided into 5 scales. The first four scales assess negative symptoms (emotional symptoms, conduct problems, hyperactivity and inattention symptoms, and peer relationship problems), while the last scale evaluates positive social relationships (prosocial behavior) [33]. Depending on the scores obtained, children are classified as normal, borderline, or abnormal. For those classified as borderline or abnormal, more in-depth studies are required to diagnose a behavioral problem. We selected this test because it is effective in differentiating between psychiatric and non-psychiatric populations, with the advantage of being shorter than other behavioral tests [34].

At the same time, we assessed the children using a BDI screening test. These results are shown in an earlier article published by our research group [29].

2.4. Statistical Analysis

A descriptive analysis was carried out to detail the frequency distribution of the different variables in the cohort, along with the distribution of the behavioral classifications in each scale. We examined the relationship between the sociodemographic variables, Doppler measurements and FGR characteristics, and the behavioral problems in each scale using the chi-squared test.

Finally, we conducted a multiple linear regression analysis to investigate the effect of (1) sociodemographic variables, (2) FGR characteristics and age at delivery, and (3) neonatal and child outcomes on the score from the total difficulties scale. Normality was tested using a Kolmogorov–Smirnov analysis. Pearson's coefficient was used for the correlations when we confirmed the normal distribution. For all analyses, we considered a p-value below 0.05 to be significant. All data were processed and analyzed with the support of the Statistical Package for the Social Sciences (SPSS), version 22.0 (SPSS Inc., Chicago, IL, USA).

3. Results

3.1. Population and Characteristics of Population Participants

One hundred and thirty children diagnosed with FGR during pregnancy who were born in 2015 were initially located. Figure 1 describes our flow diagram of the participants in the research. The study was carried out in a single medical facility; therefore, no sampling of cases was carried out. Consequently, all diagnosed cases of FGR that met the inclusion criteria were considered for the study. Seventy 6-year-old children were recruited, representing the initial population with a confidence level of 95%, a type-II error of 0.6, and a statistical power of 94% [29].

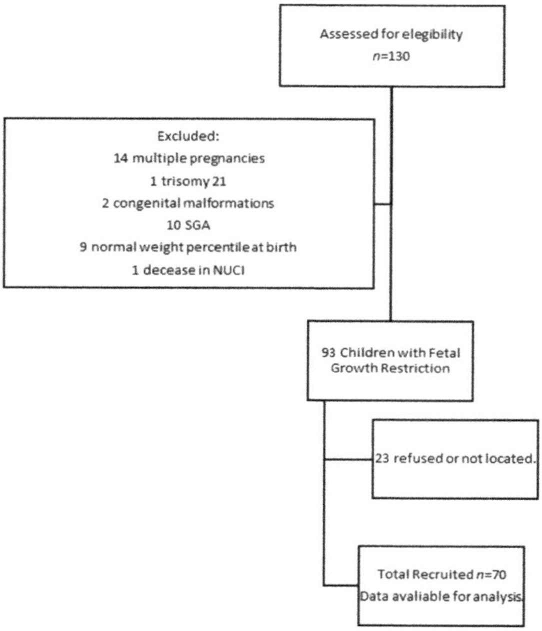

Figure 1. Flow diagram detailing the participants in the research.

The characteristics of the population participants were described in our previous paper [29]. Table 2 summarizes the sociodemographics, delivery characteristics, and adverse neonatal outcomes of the population.

Table 2. Sociodemographics, delivery characteristics, and neonatal outcome frequencies.

Variables	n (%)	Mean ± SD
Separated parents	21 (30)	
Maternal educational level		
Primary school	7 (10)	
Secondary school	38 (54.3)	
Bachelor's degree	23 (32.9)	
Paternal educational level		
Primary school	18 (25.7)	
Secondary school	36 (51.4)	
Bachelor's degree	13 (18.6)	
Maternal Unemployed status	25 (35.7)	
Paternal Unemployed status	8 (11.4)	

Table 2. *Cont.*

Variables	*n* (%)	Mean ± SD
Socioeconomic status		
Low	10 (14.3)	
Middle	54 (77.1)	
High	4 (5.7)	
Smoker in pregnancy	16 (22.9)	
Postpartum depression	14 (20)	
Pre-eclampsia	24 (34.3)	
Gestational age at diagnosis of FGR (mean)		
Early onset	23 (32.9)	33.14 ± 4.31
Late onset	46 (65.7)	
Fetal weight at diagnosis		1616.38 g ± 660.25
UA PI Percentile (mean)		61.52 ± 27.94
Pathologic	14 (20)	
MCA PI Percentile (mean)		15.69 ± 22.68
Pathologic	29 (41.4)	
CPR percentile (mean)		14.18 ± 22.74
Pathologic	35 (50)	
Vaginal delivery	25 (35.7)	
Cesarean section	45 (64.3)	
Gestational age at delivery		35.61 ± 3.21
<28 weeks	2 (2.9)	
28–32 weeks	10 (14.3)	
32–37 weeks	28 (40)	
>37 weeks	30 (42.9)	
Pathological non-stressant test	31 (44.3)	
Arterial blood cord pH		7.27 ± 0.09
Birthweight (grams)		1848.30 ± 589.74
Gender (female)	37 (52.9)	
Head circumference at delivery (cm)		30.26 ± 3.37
Breastfeeding	52 (74.3)	
Days of NICU admission		127 ± 26.78
Neonatal outcomes		
ARDS	22 (31.4)	
Neonatal sepsis	14 (20)	
ROP	6 (8.6)	
BPD	4 (5.7)	
GMH	3 (4.3)	
PDA	6 (8.6)	
NEC	3 (4.3)	
Intestinal perforation	2 (2.9)	
Acute kidney failure	2 (2.9)	

FGR: fetal growth restriction, UA PI: umbilical artery pulsatility index, MCA PI: middle cerebral artery pulsatility index, CPR: cerebroplacental ratio, SD: standard deviation, NICU: neonatal intensive care unit, ARDS: acute respiratory distress syndrome, ROP: retinopathy of prematurity, BDP: bronchopulmonary dysplasia, GMH: germinal matrix hemorrhage, PDA: patent ductus arteriosus, NEC: necrotizing enterocolitis.

3.2. Behavioral Outcomes at 6 Years of Age

The children were aged 70–84 months at the time of the behavioral test. The average age of the children at the time of assessment was 76.20 months old (SD = 3.70). The learning disabilities rate was 27.1%. Additionally, 36.8% of the children needed early child support, and 16.7% of the children are currently following this program. Parents reported two cases of children who were diagnosed as having an autistic spectrum disorder. One of these children exhibited difficulties in performing adaptive skills, while the other child exhibited a global development disorder. These data were published in our previous paper [29].

Table 3 summarizes the percentages of children with behavioral problems in different areas. We were able to record 30% of the global behavioral disabilities. In the case of hyperactivity symptoms, 30% of the children had an abnormal classification, and 8.6% had a borderline classification. Hyperactivity symptoms and conduct problems were the most common issues.

Table 3. Percentages of children with behavioral problems.

SDQ Scales	Normal (%)	Borderline (%)	Abnormal (%)
Total difficulties	70	15.7	14.3
Emotional problems	72.9	10	17.1
Conduct problems	62.9	25.7	11.4
Hyperactivity	61.4	8.6	30
Peer problems	78.6	11.4	10
Prosocial	95.7	2.9	1.4

We found a positive correlation between the total score and the scores obtained on different scales: emotional scale (r = 0.655, $p \leq 0.001$), behavior scale (r = 0.655, $p \leq 0.001$), hyperactivity (r = 0.843, $p \leq 0.001$), and peer problems (r = 0.465, $p \leq 0.001$). Similarly, a positive correlation was found between the hyperactivity and emotional scale (r = 0.387, $p = 0.001$) and the behavior scale (r = 0.549, $p \leq 0.001$). Therefore, hyperactive children tended to present more emotional and behavioral problems.

3.3. Bivariant Analyses

Tables 4 and 5 summarize the percentages of children with behavioral problems according to the diagnosis variables. We found no differences in the classification according to the onset time of FGR. However, with the exception of the peer problems scale, there was a tendency of poor results in each scale for the early-onset FGR diagnosis group. Learning difficulties were more frequent in the early-onset FGR group (43.5%) than in the late-onset FGR group (19.6%), reaching statistical significance ($\chi^2(1, N = 69) = 4.39$, $p = 0.036$).

Table 4. Percentages of children with behavior problems, depending on FGR onset.

	FGR Onset	Normal	Borderline	Abnormal	
Total	E-O	65.2	17.4	17.4	n/s
	L-O	71.7	15.2	13	
Emotional	E-O	65.2	21.7	13	n/s
	L-O	76.1	4.3	19.6	
Conduct	E-O	60.9	34.8	4.3	n/s
	L-O	63	21.7	15.2	
Hyperactivity	E-O	56.5	4.3	39.1	n/s
	L-O	63	18.9	26.1	
Peer problems	E-O	82.6	13	4.3	n/s
	L-O	76.1	10.9	13	
Prosocial	E-O	100	0	0	n/s
	L-O	93.5	4.3	2.2	

E-O: Early-onset, L-O: Late-onset, n/s: not significant.

Regarding the Doppler measurement variables, we found that a pathological CPR measurement was related to poor results on the full scale. When pathological UA, MCA, and CPR measurements were detected, there was a tendency towards poor classifications in the remaining behavioral scales (no significance).

Table 5. Percentages of children with behavioral problems, depending on Doppler measurements.

	UA	Normal (%)	Borderline (%)	Abnormal (%)	
Total	Pathological	64.3	14.3	21.4	n/s
	Normal	74.5	13.7	11.8	
Emotional	Pathological	64.3	14.3	21.4	n/s
	Normal	74.5	9.8	15.7	
Conduct	Pathological	64.3	28.6	7.1	n/s
	Normal	64.7	23.5	11.8	
Hyperactivity	Pathological	50	14.3	35.7	n/s
	Normal	66.7	7.8	25.5	
Peer problems	Pathological	78.6	14.3	7.1	n/s
	Normal	80.4	7.8	11.8	
Prosocial	Pathological	100	0	0	n/s
	Normal	94.1	3.9	2	
	MCA				
Total	Pathological	69	17.2	13.8	n/s
	Normal	80	13.3	6.7	
Emotional	Pathological	69	13.8	17.2	n/s
	Normal	80	6.7	13.3	
Conduct	Pathological	62.1	31	6.9	n/s
	Normal	70	16.7	13.3	
Hyperactivity	Pathological	65.5	6.9	27.6	n/s
	Normal	66.7	10	23.3	
Peer problems	Pathological	75.9	10.3	13.8	n/s
	Normal	83.3	10	6.7	
Prosocial	Pathological	93.1	6.9	0	n/s
	Normal	96.7	0	3.3	
	CPR				
Total	Pathological	60	22.9	17.1	$\chi^2(2, N = 70) = 6.36, p = 0.042$
	Normal	88.5	11.5	0	
Emotional	Pathological	65.7	14.3	20	n/s
	Normal	88.5	3.8	7.7	
Conduct	Pathological	60	25.7	14.3	n/s
	Normal	69.2	26.9	3.8	
Hyperactivity	Pathological	57.1	11.4	31.4	n/s
	Normal	73.1	3.8	23.1	
Peer problems	Pathological	82.9	8.6	8.6	n/s
	Normal	73.1	15.4	11.5	
Prosocial	Pathological	97.1	0	2.9	n/s
	Normal	92.3	7.7	0	

UA: umbilical artery; MCA: middle cerebral artery; CPR: cerebroplacental ratio; n/s: not significant.

Gestational age at delivery or birth characteristics were not related to behavioral outcomes. A positive correlation was found between the birth-weight percentile at delivery and the different scales: total score ($r = -0.310$, $p = 0.009$), emotional scale ($r = -0.280$, $p = 0.019$), and hyperactivity scale ($r = -0.246$, $p = 0.040$). Head circumference was not related to the results, although we were able to negatively correlate the birth-weight percentile with the score of the total scale ($r = -0.310$, $p = 0.009$), emotional scale ($r = -0.280$, $p = 0.019$), and hyperactivity scale ($r = -0.246$, $p = 0.040$). Neonatal outcome was not associated with behavioral problems.

3.4. *Multivariate Analyses*

In order to analyze the mediating factors, we performed a multiple linear regression analysis. Table 6 summarizes the variables included in each model. We included sociodemographic factors in the first model. Maternal employment status (ES) was positively related to global behavioral score ($F(1,62) = 5.15$, $p = 0.027$). In this regard, unemployed mothers had children with higher scores and, consequently, worse classifications. The R^2 value was 0.077, showing that 7% of the effect is explained by differences in the mother's ES.

Table 6. Variables included in each model.

Model	Variables
1	Separated parents Maternal and paternal educational level Maternal and paternal employment status Socioeconomic status
2	Doppler measurements: UA-PI percentile, MCA-PI percentile, and CPR percentile Birthweight percentile at delivery Gestational age at delivery
3	Gender Adverse neonatal outcomes Early child support Academic difficulties Nursery assistance

UA-PI: umbilical artery pulsatility index; MCA-PI: middle cerebral artery pulsatility index; CPR: cerebroplacental ratio.

In the second model, the birth-weight percentile was negatively related to the total score ($F(1,59) = 5.58$, $p = 0.022$) in the second model. The R^2 value was 0.089; therefore, this variable could explain the 8.9% effect.

In the third model, we found that the need for early child support was negatively related to the total score of behavioral problems ($F(1,59) = 5.22$, $p = 0.026$). These findings could be explained by the higher rates of severe FGR and extreme prematurity among these children, making them more prone to behavioral disabilities. Table 7 sums up these models.

Table 7. Multiple linear regression values of the different models.

Model	Variables	B	Standard Error	T	95% CI		*p*	R^2
					Lower	Upper		
1	Maternal employment status	−2.97	1.31	−2.26	−5.60	−0.355	0.027	0.077
	(Constant)	12.95	1.06	12.18	10.82	15.08	<0.001	
2	Birth-weight percentile	−0.659	0.279	−2.36	−1.21	−0.100	0.022	0.089
	(Constant)	11.26	0.697	16.15	9.86	12.66	<0.001	
3	Need for early child support	3.28	1.43	2.28	0.409	6.16	0.026	0.081
	(Constant)	9.6	0.781	12.3	8.04	11.16	<0.001	

Variables with significant value in the different models: maternal employment status (unemployed or active worker), birth-weight percentile, and early child support (yes or no). B: beta standardized coefficient, T: t-value, *p*: *p*-value, R^2: R-squared value, CI: confidence interval.

4. Discussion

We conducted a study to assess the behavioral development of children with FGR at 6 years of age. We have demonstrated higher behavioral disability rates in these children, specifically, high rates of hyperactivity or conduct problems. At the same time, we have proved a negative relationship between the birth-weight percentile and the total behavioral scale score.

FGR is a cause for concern among obstetricians due to the perinatal morbidities it generates, which are secondary to prematurity or the hemodynamic process itself. In recent decades, the neurodevelopmental deficits of these children, especially behavioral or cognitive impairments, have attracted the attention of both clinicians and researchers.

4.1. Regarding the Prevalence of Behavioral Disorders

Our study assessed the possible behavioral problems at the age of 6 (70–84 months) of children previously diagnosed with FGR. At this stage, the children's attentional capacity has matured to the point where they are able to maintain a state of alertness, their ability to resolve conflicts or problems has increased, and psychosocial relationships with their environment are well established.

Multiple studies have shown that the neurodevelopment of children with FGR during childhood is not comparable to that of children with a normal birth weight. In our study, we found a high prevalence of possible behavioral problems. In fact, 14.3% of the children had abnormal scores on the questionnaire, while 15.7% had borderline scores. Therefore, 30% of the children assessed (abnormal and borderline scores) should undergo more specific evaluations to establish a correct diagnosis. In particular, within the areas studied, the areas of conduct (borderline: 25.7%, abnormal: 11.4%) and hyperactivity (borderline: 8.6%, abnormal: 30%) were the most affected (externalizing problems), while emotional areas and peer problems were less strongly affected (internalizing difficulties). Parents reported that 27.1% of the children had experienced learning difficulties at school.

When evaluating these differences based on the time of FGR diagnosis, early-onset FGR presented worse scores in terms of externalizing problems (behavior and hyperactivity), while late-onset FGR presented worse scores in terms of peer problems and prosocial areas. Similarly, we found a higher percentage of academic difficulties in the subgroup of children diagnosed with early-onset FGR (43.5%) compared to children diagnosed with late-onset FGR (19.6%).

Several studies have shown similar results to ours. Guellec et al. (2011) assessed children at 8 years of age using the SDQ. They identified 33.3% of behavioral problems in FGR infants that were born before 28 weeks of gestational age and 19.1% of behavioral problems in those born between 29 and 32 weeks of gestational age. Similarly, the learning difficulties rates were similar to ours, with 35.5% in those born before 28 weeks of gestational age and 28% in those born between 29 and 32 weeks of gestational age. However, their hyperactivity problem rates varied between 19.1 and 23.5%, while we found 39.1% of hyperactivity disabilities in those children diagnosed before 32 weeks of gestation (data not shown). It is important to note that they classified and evaluated infants by gestational age in their study, without determining which subjects presented real growth restrictions [19].

A previous meta-analysis evaluated behavioral and executive function problems in infants born before 33 weeks of gestation or weighing less than 1500 g. Compared to those born at term or at an appropriate weight, the infants displayed worse results in terms of academic achievement, attention, internalizing problems, and executive function. However, the analysis did not differentiate between growth restriction and growth that was appropriate for the subjects' gestational age [14]. We must note that executive function is a cognitive process and has significant implications for behavioral skills such as self-regulation and inhibition [35].

These findings have also been supported by studies on late-onset FGR children. Geva et al. (2006) showed that FGR children presented a higher incidence of learning disabilities, memory problems, low creativity, and executive function problems compared to children with normal growth [16]. Similarly, Kulseng et al. (2007) found that children born with a very low birth weight at term (less than 1500 gr) presented worse results in terms of attention tasks and executive function at 14 years of age, at around 25% [23]. However, in another study, attention deficit and hyperactivity disorders were slightly higher in underweight children than in the normal-weight population [36]. The authors did not perform a correct discrimination of growth restriction, so it is impossible to compare their findings with those in our study. On the other hand, we did not conduct a specific evaluation of the attentional network. Despite the fact that we found a high rate of attention and hyperactivity problems in our population, a diagnostic test is needed to confirm this finding.

We did not find a relationship between the behavior assessment results and gestational age at delivery, although we did find that children with a lower birth weight had poor results regarding the total, emotional, and hyperactivity scores. This may be due to our sample size. Nevertheless, a previous meta-analysis found that being underweight and premature may lead to attention-deficit hyperactivity disorders [37].

Behavioral disabilities have significant consequences since problems in this area in the preschool years may be associated with a higher prevalence of externalizing and internalizing problems at the age of 10–14 years, leading to learning and adaptation problems [38].

4.2. Regarding the Prediction of Doppler Markers and Prematurity

Doppler markers have proven useful in monitoring FGR fetuses to reduce perinatal morbidity and mortality. The umbilical artery (UA) has been the major protagonist in predicting short-term adverse outcomes in this group of children [39–41]. However, associations between the changes in UA waves and neurodevelopment, specifically psychosocial and academic development, are controversial [42,43]. In our case, when we evaluated the predictive capacity of the UA in neurodevelopment, we found no association between its percentile and the results on the SDQ, so we could not relate it to behavioral effects. Nonetheless, children with a pathological pulsatility index (PI) for the UA tended to present worse outcomes. These results must be interpreted with caution since we have only a few cases of extreme prematurity and pathological UA waves.

Traditionally, brain sparing has been considered a protective factor to maintain proper brain function in more critical hemodynamic situations. However, this fact is controversial, and multiple studies have shown that it may not entirely be a protective factor. Regarding behavior, Richter et al. (2020) found that the presence of brain sparing was associated with better behavioral outcomes, specifically externalized behavioral profiles (conduct and hyperactivity) [44]. Other studies have failed to link this phenomenon to behavioral issues when assessing children later [45,46]. However, the parents reported more socialization and attention problems in children that had shown brain sparing, although this was not verified with diagnostic tests [45]. In our case, we observed in the bivariate analysis that those children with a pathological CPR had significantly worse scores on the total behavior scale. Emotional, conduct, and hyperactivity areas were also negatively affected by brain sparing, although the values did not reach significance.

The brain-sparing effect has been confirmed by several studies as a hierarchy process, such that when vasodilation is detected in the middle cerebral artery (MCA), this process has already occurred in the anterior cerebral artery (ACA). This hierarchy has been associated with poorer cognitive outcomes, specifically in terms of attention, social interaction, and adaptation abilities [47]. In our case, due to the design of our study, we were not able to verify this hierarchy. However, we observed that children who presented a brain-sparing process (whether by a pathological MCA or CPR) had a higher rate of psychosocial and hyperactivity symptoms.

Despite the importance of redistribution, gestational age at delivery remains the main factor regarding neurological development during childhood [45,48,49]. Nevertheless, the severity of growth restriction may be a risk marker for the appearance of behavioral problems during childhood and adolescence, and, thus, may inform future screening and prevention strategies.

Our study has several strengths. The most important of these is the strict definition of the FGR condition. This allows us not to underestimate our results. Moreover, we have carried out an assessment of children at a late age (6 years of age). At this age, social skills and behavioral problems are well established. Finally, we assessed the children using the SDQ, a validated screening test that allows for the correct discrimination between pathological and non-pathological cases [32,34].

Our main limitation was the sample size. As a single-center study, we were unable to locate a large number of children with a history of FGR. Of those cases that were found, a small proportion of parents could not be located or refused to be assessed. Because of our small sample size, the R-square coefficient obtained was low, this being a limitation in our multiple linear regression model. It would explain the low percentage of variability obtained. Furthermore, we could not evaluate a control group without growth restriction to compare the results obtained. Although the behavioral assessment was prospective, the cohort design was retrospective. This fact only provides an association between behavioral outcomes and FGR characteristics. A multicenter study with a larger sample size and a control group is needed in order to verify our findings.

5. Conclusions

We found high behavioral disability rates, particularly in the hyperactivity or conduct areas, in children with FGR. At the same time, we found a negative relationship between the birth-weight percentile and the score of the total behavioral scale. Regarding FGR onset, early-onset FGR children presented poor scores for externalizing problems (behavior and hyperactivity), while late-onset FGR children presented worse scores regarding problems with peers and prosocial areas. No relationship was found between gestational age at delivery and behavioral disabilities. Behavior was not affected by gestational age at delivery, although it was influenced by birth weight. However, the hyperactivity scale was not affected by either birth weight or gestational age at delivery. We observed that children exhibiting brain sparing presented significantly worse results in the total behavior scale, in addition to a negative effect in the emotional, conduct, and hyperactivity areas.

Author Contributions: Conceptualization, M.J.B.M. and E.G.M.; methodology, M.J.B.M. and E.G.M.; software, M.J.B.M.; validation, E.G.M.; formal analysis, M.J.B.M. and E.G.M.; investigation, M.J.B.M. and E.G.M.; resources, M.B.A.; data curation, M.J.B.M. and E.G.M.; writing—original draft preparation, M.J.B.M. and M.B.A.; writing—review and editing, M.J.B.M., M.B.A. and E.G.M.; visualization, M.J.B.M., M.B.A. and E.G.M.; supervision, E.G.M. All authors have read and agreed to the published version of the manuscript.

Funding: This research received no external funding. Málaga University supported publication charges.

Institutional Review Board Statement: The study was conducted in accordance with the Declaration of Helsinki and approved by the Ethics Committee of the "Comité de Etica de Investigación Provincial de Málaga" (28 January 2021).

Informed Consent Statement: Informed consent was obtained from all subjects involved in the study.

Data Availability Statement: Not applicable.

Acknowledgments: The authors would like to thank all the participants in this study and Malaga University for their support.

Conflicts of Interest: The authors declare no conflict of interest.

References

1. Figueras, F.; Gratacós, E. Update on the Diagnosis and Classification of Fetal Growth Restriction and Proposal of a Stage-Based Management Protocol. *Fetal Diagn. Ther.* **2014**, *36*, 86–98. [CrossRef]
2. Lees, C.; Marlow, N.; Arabin, B.; Bilardo, C.M.; Brezinka, C.; Derks, J.B.; Duvekot, J.; Frusca, T.; Diemert, A.; Ferrazzi, E.; et al. Perinatal morbidity and mortality in early-onset fetal growth restriction: Cohort outcomes of the trial of randomized umbilical and fetal flow in Europe (TRUFFLE). *Ultrasound Obstet. Gynecol.* **2013**, *42*, 400–408. [CrossRef] [PubMed]
3. Thornton, J.G.; Hornbuckle, J.; Vail, A.; Spiegelhalter, D.J.; Levene, M.; GRIT study group. Infant wellbeing at 2 years of age in the Growth Restriction Intervention Trial (GRIT): Multicentred randomised controlled trial. *Lancet* **2004**, *364*, 513–520. [PubMed]
4. Costeloe, K.L.; Hennessy, E.M.; Haider, S.; Stacey, F.; Marlow, N.; Draper, E.S. Short term outcomes after extreme preterm birth in England: Comparison of two birth cohorts in 1995 and 2006 (the EPICure studies). *BMJ* **2012**, *345*, e7976. [CrossRef] [PubMed]
5. Simeoni, U.; Armengaud, J.-B.; Siddeek, B.; Tolsa, J.-F. Perinatal Origins of Adult Disease. *Neonatology* **2018**, *113*, 393–399. [CrossRef]
6. Padilla, N.; Perapoch, J.; Carrascosa, A.; Acosta-Rojas, R.; Botet, F.; Gratacós, E. Twelve-month neurodevelopmental outcome in preterm infants with and without intrauterine growth restriction. *Acta Paediatr.* **2010**, *99*, 1498–1503. [CrossRef]
7. Samuelsen, G.B.; Pakkenberg, B.; Bogdanović, N.; Gundersen, H.J.G.; Larsen, J.F.; Græm, N.; Laursen, H. Severe cell reduction in the future brain cortex in human growth–restricted fetuses and infants. *Am. J. Obstet. Gynecol.* **2007**, *197*, 56.e1–56.e7. [CrossRef]

8. Tolsa, C.B.; Zimine, S.; Warfield, S.K.; Freschi, M.; Rossignol, A.S.; Lazeyras, F.; Hanquinet, S.; Pfizenmaier, M.; Hüppi, P.S. Early Alteration of Structural and Functional Brain Development in Premature Infants Born with Intrauterine Growth Restriction. *Pediatr. Res.* **2004**, *56*, 132–138. [CrossRef]
9. Mallard, C.; Loeliger, M.; Copolov, D.; Rees, S. Reduced number of neurons in the hippocampus and the cerebellum in the postnatal guinea-pig following intrauterine growth-restriction. *Neuroscience* **2000**, *100*, 327–333. [CrossRef]
10. Bruno, C.J.; Bengani, S.; Gomes, W.A.; Brewer, M.; Vega, M.; Xie, X.; Kim, M.; Fuloria, M. MRI Differences Associated with Intrauterine Growth Restriction in Preterm Infants. *Neonatology* **2017**, *111*, 317–323. [CrossRef]
11. Fischi-Gómez, E.; Vasung, L.; Meskaldji, D.-E.; Lazeyras, F.; Borradori-Tolsa, C.; Hagmann, P.; Barisnikov, K.; Thiran, J.-P.; Hüppi, P.S. Structural Brain Connectivity in School-Age Preterm Infants Provides Evidence for Impaired Networks Relevant for Higher Order Cognitive Skills and Social Cognition. *Cereb. Cortex* **2015**, *25*, 2793–2805. [CrossRef] [PubMed]
12. Padilla, N.; Junqué, C.; Figueras, F.; Sanz-Cortes, M.; Bargalló, N.; Arranz, A.; Donaire, A.; Figueras, J.; Gratacos, E. Differential vulnerability of gray matter and white matter to intrauterine growth restriction in preterm infants at 12 months corrected age. *Brain Res.* **2014**, *1545*, 1–11. [CrossRef] [PubMed]
13. Dubois, J.; Benders, M.; Borradori-Tolsa, C.; Cachia, A.; Lazeyras, F.; Ha-Vinh Leuchter, R.; Sizonenko, S.V.; Warfield, S.K.; Mangin, J.F.; Hüppi, P.S. Primary cortical folding in the human newborn: An early marker of later functional development. *Brain* **2008**, *131*, 2028–2041. [CrossRef] [PubMed]
14. Aarnoudse-Moens, C.S.H.; Weisglas-Kuperus, N.; van Goudoever, J.B.; Oosterlaan, J. Meta-Analysis of Neurobehavioral Outcomes in Very Preterm and/or Very Low Birth Weight Children. *Pediatrics* **2009**, *124*, 717–728. [CrossRef]
15. Arpino, C.; Compagnone, E.; Montanaro, M.L.; Cacciatore, D.; De Luca, A.; Cerulli, A.; Di Girolamo, S.; Curatolo, P. Preterm birth and neurodevelopmental outcome: A review. *Child's Nerv. Syst.* **2010**, *26*, 1139–1149. [CrossRef]
16. Geva, R.; Eshel, R.; Leitner, Y.; Valevski, A.F.; Harel, S. Neuropsychological Outcome of Children with Intrauterine Growth Restriction: A 9-Year Prospective Study. *Pediatrics* **2006**, *118*, 91–100. [CrossRef]
17. Geva, R.; Eshel, R.; Leitner, Y.; Fattal-Valevski, A.; Harel, S. Memory functions of children born with asymmetric intrauterine growth restriction. *Brain Res.* **2006**, *1117*, 186–194. [CrossRef]
18. Gortner, L.; van Husen, M.; Thyen, U.; Gembruch, U.; Friedrich, H.-J.; Landmann, E. Outcome in preterm small for gestational age infants compared to appropriate for gestational age preterms at the age of 2 years: A prospective study. *Eur. J. Obstet. Gynecol. Reprod. Biol.* **2003**, *110*, S93–S97. [CrossRef]
19. Guellec, I.; Lapillonne, A.; Renolleau, S.; Charlaluk, M.-L.; Roze, J.-C.; Marret, S.; Vieux, R.; Monique, K.; Ancel, P.-Y.; The EPIPAGE Study Group. Neurologic Outcomes at School Age in Very Preterm Infants Born with Severe or Mild Growth Restriction. *Pediatrics* **2011**, *127*, e883–e891. [CrossRef]
20. Morsing, E.; Asard, M.; Ley, D.; Stjernqvist, K.; Marsal, K. Cognitive Function After Intrauterine Growth Restriction and Very Preterm Birth. *Pediatrics* **2011**, *127*, e874–e882. [CrossRef]
21. Arcangeli, T.; Thilaganathan, B.; Hooper, R.; Khan, K.S.; Bhide, A. Neurodevelopmental delay in small babies at term: A systematic review. *Ultrasound Obstet. Gynecol.* **2012**, *40*, 267–275. [CrossRef]
22. De Bie, H.M.A.; Oostrom, K.J.; Delemarre-van de Waal, H.A. Brain Development, Intelligence and Cognitive Outcome in Children Born Small for Gestational Age. *Horm. Res. Paediatr.* **2010**, *73*, 6–14. [CrossRef]
23. Kulseng, S.; Jennekens-Schinkel, A.; Naess, P.; Romundstad, P.; Indredavik, M.; Vik, T.; Brubakk, A.M. Very-low-birthweight and term small-for-gestational-age adolescents: Attention revisited. *Acta Paediatr.* **2007**, *95*, 224–230. [CrossRef]
24. Paz, I.; Laor, A.; Gale, R.; Harlap, S.; Stevenson, D.K.; Seidman, D.S. Term infants with fetal growth restriction are not at increased risk for low intelligence scores at age 17 years. *J. Pediatr.* **2001**, *138*, 87–91. [CrossRef]
25. Savchev, S.; Sanz-Cortes, M.; Cruz-Martinez, R.; Arranz, A.; Botet, F.; Gratacos, E.; Figueras, F. Neurodevelopmental outcome of full-term small-for-gestational-age infants with normal placental function. *Ultrasound Obstet. Gynecol.* **2013**, *42*, 201–206. [CrossRef] [PubMed]
26. Sommerfelt, K. Cognitive development of term small for gestational age children at five years of age. *Arch. Dis. Child.* **2000**, *83*, 25–30. [CrossRef] [PubMed]
27. Theodore, R.F.; Thompson, J.M.D.; Waldie, K.E.; Becroft, D.M.O.; Robinson, E.; Wild, C.J.; Clark, P.M.; Mitchell, E.A.; Wild, C. Determinants of cognitive ability at 7 years: A longitudinal case–control study of children born small-for-gestational age at term. *Eur. J. Pediatr.* **2009**, *168*, 1217–1224. [CrossRef] [PubMed]
28. Benítez-Marín, M.J.; Marín-Clavijo, J.; Blanco-Elena, J.A.; Jiménez-López, J.; González-Mesa, E. Brain Sparing Effect on Neurodevelopment in Children with Intrauterine Growth Restriction: A Systematic Review. *Children* **2021**, *8*, 745. [CrossRef]
29. Benítez Marín, M.J.; Blanco Elena, J.A.; Marín Clavijo, J.; Jiménez López, J.; Lubián López, D.M.; González Mesa, E. Neurodevelopment Outcome in Children with Fetal Growth Restriction at Six Years of Age: A Retrospective Cohort Study. *Int. J. Environ. Res. Public Health* **2022**, *19*, 11043. [CrossRef]
30. Spittle, A.; Orton, J.; Anderson, P.J.; Boyd, R.; Doyle, L.W. Early developmental intervention programmes provided post hospital discharge to prevent motor and cognitive impairment in preterm infants. *Cochrane Database Syst. Rev.* **2015**, *2015*, CD005495. [CrossRef]
31. Robert Goodman. Available online: https://www.sdqinfo.org/a0.html (accessed on 1 December 2020).
32. Goodman, R. The Strengths and Difficulties Questionnaire: A Research Note. *J. Child Psychol. Psychiatry* **1997**, *38*, 581–586. [CrossRef] [PubMed]

33. Goodman, R. The Extended Version of the Strengths and Difficulties Questionnaire as a Guide to Child Psychiatric Caseness and Consequent Burden. *J. Child Psychol. Psychiatry* **1999**, *40*, 791–799. [CrossRef] [PubMed]
34. Español-Martín, G.; Pagerols, M.; Prat, R.; Rivas, C.; Sixto, L.; Valero, S.; Artigas, M.S.; Ribasés, M.; Ramos-Quiroga, J.A.; Casas, M.; et al. Strengths and Difficulties Questionnaire: Psychometric Properties and Normative Data for Spanish 5- to 17-Year-Olds. *Assessment* **2021**, *28*, 1445–1458. [CrossRef]
35. Duncan, A.F.; Matthews, M.A. Neurodevelopmental Outcomes in Early Childhood. *Clin. Perinatol.* **2018**, *45*, 377–392. [CrossRef] [PubMed]
36. Indredavik, M.S.; Vik, T.; Heyerdahl, S.; Kulseng, S.; Fayers, P.; Brubakk, A.M. Psychiatric symptoms and disorders in adolescents with low birth weight. *Arch. Dis. Child-Fetal Neonatal Ed.* **2004**, *89*, F445–F450. [CrossRef] [PubMed]
37. Franz, A.P.; Bolat, G.U.; Bolat, H.; Matijasevich, A.; Santos, I.S.; Silveira, R.C.; Procianoy, R.S.; Rohde, L.A.; Moreira-Maia, C.R. Attention-Deficit/Hyperactivity Disorder and Very Preterm/Very Low Birth Weight: A Meta-analysis. *Pediatrics* **2018**, *141*, e20171645. [CrossRef]
38. Bornstein, M.H.; Hahn, C.-S.; Haynes, O.M. Social competence, externalizing, and internalizing behavioral adjustment from early childhood through early adolescence: Developmental cascades. *Dev. Psychopathol.* **2010**, *22*, 717–735. [CrossRef]
39. Valcamonico, A.; Danti, L.; Frusca, T.; Soregaroli, M.; Zucca, S.; Abrami, F.; Tiberti, A. Absent end-diastolic velocity in umbilical artery: Risk of neonatal morbidity and brain damage. *Am. J. Obstet. Gynecol.* **1994**, *170*, 796–801. [CrossRef]
40. Voßbeck, S.; de Camargo, O.K.; Grab, D.; Bode, H.; Pohlandt, F. Neonatal and neurodevelopmental outcome in infants born before 30 weeks of gestation with absent or reversed end-diastolic flow velocities in the umbilical artery. *Eur. J. Pediatr.* **2001**, *160*, 128–134. [CrossRef]
41. Soregaroli, M.; Bonera, R.; Danti, L.; Dinolfo, D.; Taddei, F.; Valcamonico, A.; Frusca, T. Prognostic role of umbilical artery Doppler velocimetry in growth-restricted fetuses. *J. Matern. Fetal Neonatal Med.* **2002**, *11*, 199–203. [CrossRef]
42. Kirsten, G.F.; van Zyl, J.I.; van Zijl, F.; Maritz, J.S.; Odendaal, H.J. Infants of Women with Severe Early Pre-Eclampsia: The Effect of Absent End-Diastolic Umbilical Artery Doppler Flow Velocities on Neurodevelopmental Outcome. *Obstet. Gynecol. Surv.* **2001**, *56*, 124–125. [CrossRef]
43. Schreuder, A.M. Outcome at school age following antenatal detection of absent or reversed end diastolic flow velocity in the umbilical artery. *Arch. Dis. Child-Fetal Neonatal Ed.* **2002**, *86*, F108–F114. [CrossRef] [PubMed]
44. Richter, A.E.; Salavati, S.; Kooi, E.M.W.; Heijer, A.E.d.; Foreman, A.B.; Schoots, M.H.; Bilardo, C.M.; Scherjon, S.A.; Tanis, J.C.; Bos, A.F. Fetal Brain-Sparing, Postnatal Cerebral Oxygenation, and Neurodevelopment at 4 Years of Age Following Fetal Growth Restriction. *Front. Pediatr.* **2020**, *8*, 225. [CrossRef] [PubMed]
45. Beukers, F.; Aarnoudse-Moens, C.S.H.; van Weissenbruch, M.M.; Ganzevoort, W.; van Goudoever, J.B.; van Wassenaer-Leemhuis, A.G. Fetal Growth Restriction with Brain Sparing: Neurocognitive and Behavioral Outcomes at 12 Years of Age. *J. Pediatr.* **2017**, *188*, 103–109. [CrossRef] [PubMed]
46. Van den Broek, A.J.M.; Kok, J.H.; Houtzager, B.A.; Scherjon, S.A. Behavioural problems at the age of eleven years in preterm-born children with or without fetal brain sparing: A prospective cohort study. *Early Hum. Dev.* **2010**, *86*, 379–384. [CrossRef]
47. Hernandez-Andrade, E.; Figueroa-Diesel, H.; Jansson, T.; Rangel-Nava, H.; Gratacos, E. Changes in regional fetal cerebral blood flow perfusion in relation to hemodynamic deterioration in severely growth-restricted fetuses. *Ultrasound Obstet. Gynecol.* **2008**, *32*, 71–76. [CrossRef]
48. Scherjon, S.A.; Oosting, H.; Smolders-DeHaas, H.; Zondervan, H.A.; Kok, J.H. Neurodevelopmental outcome at three years of age after fetal 'brain-sparing'. *Early Hum. Dev.* **1998**, *52*, 67–79. [CrossRef]
49. Stampalija, T.; Arabin, B.; Wolf, H.; Bilardo, C.M.; Lees, C.; Brezinka, C.; Derks, J.B.; Diemert, A.; Duvekot, J.J.; Ferrazzi, E.; et al. Is middle cerebral artery Doppler related to neonatal and 2-year infant outcome in early fetal growth restriction? *Am. J. Obstet. Gynecol.* **2017**, *216*, 521.e1–521.e13. [CrossRef]

children

MDPI

Article

Use of Pulse Oximetry during Resuscitation of 230 Newborns—A Video Analysis

Vilde Kolstad [1], Hanne Pike [2], Joar Eilevstjønn [3], Frederikke Buskov [1], Hege Ersdal [4] and Siren Rettedal [1,4,*]

1 Department of Research, Stavanger University Hospital, 4019 Stavanger, Norway; vilde.hagensen.kolstad@sus.no (V.K.); frederikke.heinz.buskov@sus.no (F.B.)
2 Department of Paediatrics, Stavanger University Hospital, 4019 Stavanger, Norway; hanne.markhus.pike@sus.no
3 Laerdal Medical, 4007 Stavanger, Norway; joar.eilevstjonn@laerdal.com
4 Faculty of Health Sciences, University of Stavanger, 4021 Stavanger, Norway; hege.ersdal@safer.net
* Correspondence: siren.irene.rettedal@sus.no; Tel.: +47-4523-5742

Abstract: Background: European guidelines recommend the use of pulse oximetry (PO) during newborn resuscitation, especially when there is a need for positive pressure ventilation or supplemental oxygen. The objective was to evaluate (i) to what extent PO was used, (ii) the time and resources spent on the application of PO, and (iii) the proportion of time with a useful PO signal during newborn resuscitation. Methods: A prospective observational study was conducted at Stavanger University Hospital, Norway, between 6 June 2019 and 16 November 2021. Newborn resuscitations were video recorded, and the use of PO during the first ten minutes of resuscitation was recorded and analysed. Results: Of 7466 enrolled newborns, 289 (3.9%) received ventilation at birth. The resuscitation was captured on video in 230 cases, and these newborns were included in the analysis. PO was applied in 222 of 230 (97%) newborns, median (quartiles) 60 (24, 58) seconds after placement on the resuscitation table. The proportion of time used on application and adjustments of PO during ongoing ventilation and during the first ten minutes on the resuscitation table was 30% and 17%, respectively. Median two healthcare providers were involved in the PO application. Video of the PO monitor signal was available in 118 (53%) of the 222 newborns. The proportion of time with a useful PO signal during ventilation and during the first ten minutes on the resuscitation table was 5% and 35%, respectively. Conclusion: In total, 97% of resuscitated newborns had PO applied, in line with resuscitation guidelines. However, the application of PO was time-consuming, and a PO signal was only obtained 5% of the time during positive pressure ventilation.

Keywords: pulse oximetry; newborn saturation; heart rate assessment; heart rate monitoring; neonatal resuscitation; newborn resuscitation; resuscitation guidelines; positive pressure ventilation; NeoBeat

1. Introduction

Approximately 5% of newborns require resuscitation with positive pressure ventilations (PPV) at birth [1–4]. According to resuscitation guidelines, heart rate (HR) should be assessed after birth to evaluate the transition and identify newborns in need of resuscitation [5]. PPV should be initiated within 60 s if the newborn has not established effective breathing and HR is <100 beats per minute (bpm) and not increasing in response to initial drying and stimulation. Auscultation by stethoscope is an inexpensive and simple method that provides a rapid and intermittent assessment of HR, but HR is sometimes underestimated [2,6]. Continuous monitoring with pulse oximetry (PO) $\pm$ electrocardiogram (ECG) has the advantage of providing a more dynamic indication of HR changes and information on the responses to resuscitative interventions [5]. Several studies have shown that ECG presents HR more rapidly than PO, and that PO may underestimate HR in the initial minutes [7–12]. The Consensus on Science with Treatment Recommendations (CoSTR) from the International Liaison Committee on Resuscitation (ILCOR) therefore recommend the use of ECG for newborn HR assessment during delivery room resuscitation whenever possible [3,5]. Where ECG is not available, HR assessment with PO is a reasonable alternative, but the limitations should be kept in mind.

ECG does not replace the need for PO for evaluation of oxygenation and subsequent titration of oxygen to avoid hyper- and hypoxia [2,11]. International guidelines recommend the use of PO during PPV or when providing supplemental oxygen [2,3], and PO is common practice during newborn resuscitation in many high-resource settings [13].

The objectives were to evaluate (i) to what extent PO was used during newborn resuscitations; (ii) the number of healthcare providers (HCPs) involved, the number of single-use sensors required for the application of PO, time spent on application or adjustments of PO; and (iii) the proportion of time with a PO signal during provision of positive pressure ventilation at birth.

2. Materials and Methods

2.1. Setting

A prospective observational study was conducted at Stavanger University Hospital, Norway from 6 June 2019 to 16 November 2021. The hospital is well suited for population-based studies, being the only hospital in the region with obstetric and neonatal services and 4200 annual deliveries. Vaginal births take place in the labour ward and the midwife-run low-risk ward, and the caesarean sections in the operating theatre. PPV is provided to 3.6% of newborns, mainly by flow-driven t-piece resuscitator (NeoPuff, Fischer and Paykel, Auckland, New Zealand), alternatively a self-inflating silicone resuscitator (Laerdal, Stavanger, Norway) [4]. The paediatric resident and midwife initiate anticipated resuscitations, with the addition of a neonatologist, neonatal nurse, and an anaesthetic team for advanced resuscitations. The national resuscitation guidelines derive from the European Resuscitation Council Guidelines [2].

2.2. Data Collection and Equipment

Video recordings of resuscitations were obtained passively using motion-triggered cameras placed above the resuscitation tables, capturing the newborn and the hands of the HCPs. Dry-electrode ECG (NeoBeat, Laerdal Medical, Stavanger, Norway) was placed on the chest or upper abdomen of the newborn by the midwife assistants as soon as possible after birth. NeoBeat displays and stores HR within seconds of birth and provide continuous HR measurements. If a newborn required PPV, the cord was clamped and cut, and the newborn was carried to the resuscitation table. HCPs were instructed to apply 3-lead gel-electrode ECG (CareFusion, San Diego, CA, USA) on the newborns' chest and PO (Massimo LNCS Neo wraparound sensor, Massimo, Irvine, CA, USA) on the newborns' right hand or wrist. The order of ECG and PO placement was left to the discretion of the HCPs. However, in anticipated events, one HCP was assigned the task of applying the PO sensor. The monitor used was Carescape Patient monitor B450 or B650 (GE Healthcare, Boston, MA, USA). Video recordings were used to evaluate the time from birth to the start of ventilation, duration of PPV, application of PO and ECG, and to detect HR and PO signals displayed on the monitor. Extraction of patient characteristics were automated from electronic medical records.

2.3. Inclusion Criteria

Parents were informed and consented to participation during routine follow up in pregnancy. Newborns born at gestational age (GA) $\geq$ 28 weeks who required resuscitation with PPV at birth with the resuscitation captured on video, were enrolled.

2.4. Calculations and Definitions

All videos were manually reviewed by independent researchers (V.K. and S.R. or H.P.). Timelines were started when the newborn was placed on the resuscitation table, and for a duration of ten minutes. Videos were annotated using the ELAN 5.8 tool (The Language

Archive, Nijmegen, The Netherlands). The start of PPV was defined as when the first inflation was provided. The duration of PPV was defined as the time difference between the first and last inflation. The number of HCPs involved in applying the PO equipment and the number of single-use PO sensors used were recorded. The time spent applying the PO was defined from when one started drying the skin or picking up the sensor, whichever came first, until the PO was attached, regardless of whether a useful signal was obtained. The PO adjustment time included repositioning or reapplying the sensor, reattaching the PO cord to the monitor and/or changing the sensor. The PO signal was annotated based on reviewing a recording of the monitor screen. The time to reliable PO signal was defined as the time when a continuous pulse wave, HR, and/or saturation values were displayed for at least 3 s [7,12,14].

2.5. Statistical Analysis

Data and annotations were extracted and analysed using Matlab R2022b (MathWorks Inc., Natick, MA, USA). Continuous variables are expressed as median (quartiles) or count (%).

2.6. Ethical Considerations

This study was a part of the Safer Births Stavanger research project on newborn resuscitation, with ethical approval from the Norwegian regional ethical committee 27 April 2018 (ref.2018/338).

3. Results

In total, 10,539 newborns were born during the study period, of which 10,503 with gestational age ≥28 weeks. Of these, 7466 (71%) parents agreed to participation, of which 289 (3.9%) received PPV at birth. The resuscitation was captured on video in 230/289 cases, and these newborns were included in the analysis. A flow diagram of over participants and patient characteristics is shown in Figure 1 and Table 1, respectively.

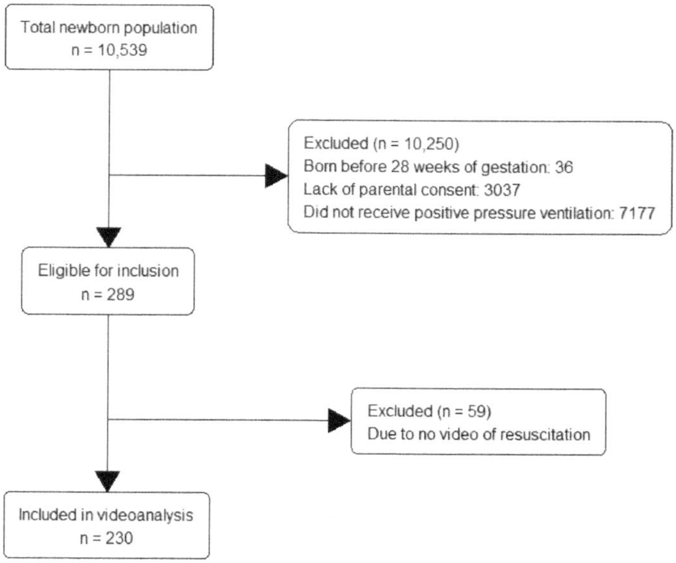

Figure 1. A flow diagram of over participants.

Table 1. Characteristics of 230 newborns included in the analysis. Characteristics are reported as median (quartiles) or count (%).

Newborn Characteristics n = 230	
Variable	
Gestational age (weeks)	40 (38, 40)
Very preterm (28 to <32 weeks)	5 (2.2%)
Moderate preterm (32 to <34 weeks)	7 (3.0%)
Late preterm (34 to <37 weeks)	21 (9.1%)
Term (≥37 weeks)	197 (85.7%)
Weight (grams)	3565 (3042, 3914)
Female gender n (%)	100 (44%)
Apgar	
1 min Apgar	5 (4, 7)
5 min Apgar	8 (6, 9)
10 min Apgar	9 (8, 10)
Umbilical cord values	
Arterial pH (*n* = 184)	7.20 (7.11, 7.25)
Arterial base excess (*n* = 176)	4.34 (1.67, 6.13)
Arterial pCO2 (*n* = 175)	8.16 (7.14, 9.64)
Pulse oximetry *n* (%)	222 (97%)
Positive pressure ventilation duration (seconds)	126 (65, 232)

3.1. Use of Auscultation, ECG and PO Assessment during Resuscitation

Among 230 resuscitated newborns, 222 (97%) had PO applied during the first 10 min on the resuscitation table. PO was applied median (quartiles) 60 (24, 58) seconds after placement on the resuscitation table.

Auscultation with the stethoscope was performed in 211 (92%) median 39 (10, 110) seconds after placement on the table.

ECG was applied in 220 (96%) newborns. Standard 3-lead gel-electrode ECG was placed in 192 newborns at a median of 60 (41, 109) seconds. Dry-electrode ECG was in most instances placed in the delivery room, and the time of placement of NeoBeat was therefore median 0 (0, 3) seconds from placement on the resuscitation table (*n* = 204).

3.2. Number of HCPs Involved and Equipment Used for Application and Adjustment of PO

For 40% of newborns, one HCP was involved in the placement of PO. For 32% and 22% of newborns, two and three HCPs were involved, respectively. For the remaining 6%, four to six HCPs were at some time involved in the placement of PO. In 82% of the 222 resuscitations, one single-use sensor was used, whereas two sensors were used in the remaining 18% of cases.

3.3. Time Spent on the Application and Adjustment of PO

The median time to start the application of PO was 60 (23, 118) seconds after the newborn was placed on the resuscitation table. Time spent on applying and adjusting PO in the first 10 min of resuscitation was median 99 (44, 223) seconds. The time spent placing the PO is illustrated in blue lines in Figure 2. The proportion of time used on application and adjustments of PO during PPV and during the first ten minutes was 30% and 17%, respectively. In 58 (26%) newborns assessed with PO, the application was not completed by the time PPV ended.

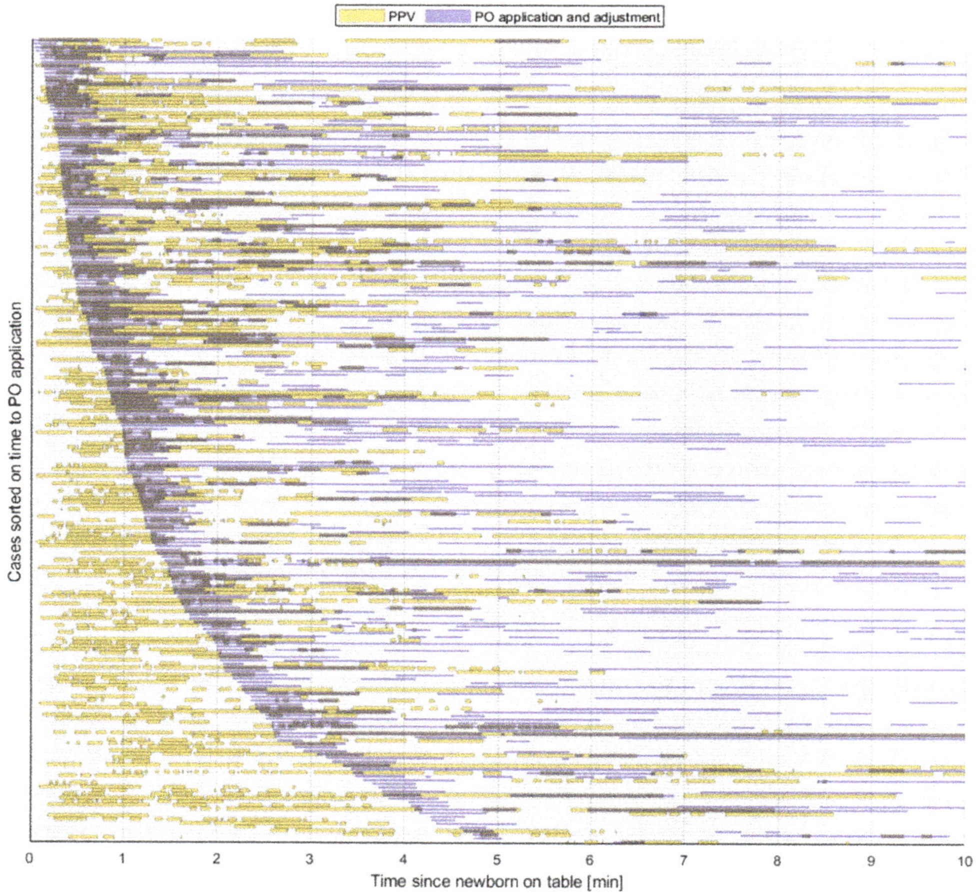

Figure 2. The figure shows 222 newborns that received PPV at birth and had PO applied. Each horizontal line represents a newborn from the time of placement on the resuscitation table (time = 0) and the first consecutive ten minutes. Provision of PPV is illustrated in orange lines. Application and/or adjustment of PO is illustrated in blue lines. Newborns are sorted by time from placement on the resuscitation table to start application of PO. PPV = positive pressure ventilation, PO = pulse oximetry.

3.4. Feedback on PO Signal

Video of the PO monitor signal was available in 118 (53%) of the 222 newborns. In 110 of 118 newborns a PO signal was obtained within the first ten minutes on the resuscitation table. The time when a PO signal was first displayed and the proportion of time with a PO signal in relation to PPV is shown in Figure 3a and b, respectively. The median time to obtain PO signal was 238 (129, 324) seconds. PPV started a median of 21 (11, 51) seconds after placement on the resuscitation table, and lasted for a duration of 126 (65, 232) seconds (data available for 222 newborns). In 85 of 118 of newborns, PO was applied during PPV. Among these, a median time with a PO signal displayed during the provision of PPV was 9 (0, 84) seconds. The proportion of time with a PO signal during PPV and during the first ten minutes after placement on the resuscitation table was 5% (0%, 31%) and 35% (9%, 49%), respectively.

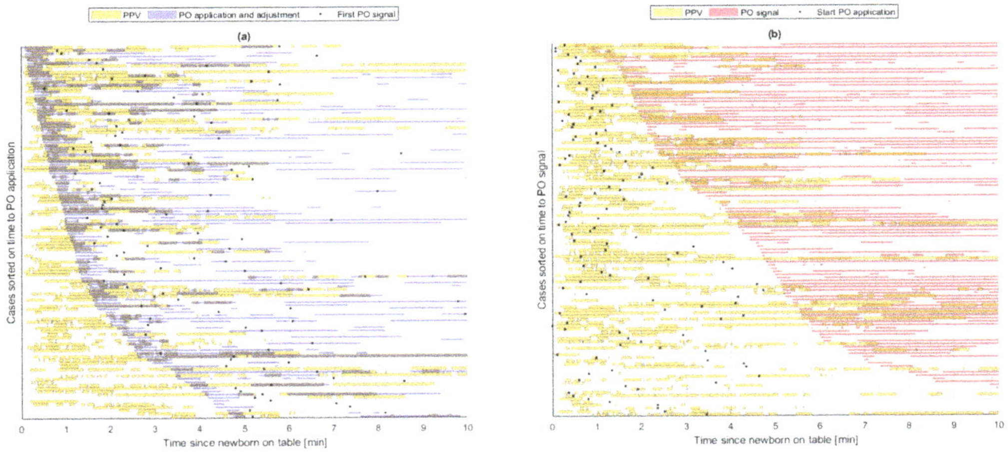

Figure 3. The figure shows the 118 newborns where video of the PO monitor was available. Each horizontal line represents a newborn from the time of placement on the resuscitation table and throughout the first ten minutes. (**a**) shows the application and adjustment of PO illustrated in blue lines in relation to PPV in orange lines, and time when the first PO signal was displayed illustrated as a black dot. (**b**) shows the proportion of time with a PO signal illustrated in pink lines in relation to PPV illustrated in orange lines. The black dot represents the start of PO application. PPV = positive pressure ventilation, PO = pulse oximetry.

4. Discussion

In this population-based video study of 230 newborns receiving PPV at birth, we found that PO was applied in 97% of resuscitations, in line with guideline recommendations [2,5]. However, HCPs spent 30% of the active resuscitation with PPV applying and adjusting the PO sensor, and median two HCPs were involved. Throughout the duration of PPV, a PO signal was only displayed 5% of the time.

An accurate HR assessment is considered important to evaluate the newborn condition, to guide management, and to evaluate the effect of resuscitative interventions. PO has several limitations with regard to monitoring HR in the delivery room. Our group has recently shown that PO displayed HR values later and for a shorter proportion of newborn resuscitation, when compared to the dry-electrode ECG device NeoBeat or standard three-lead ECG [15]. PO may furthermore underestimate HR signal for the first five to six minutes during newborn transition or resuscitation, especially in the more compromised newborns [12,15–17].

In the current study, the median time to obtain a PO signal was 237 s after placement on the resuscitation table. Similar findings have been reported previously, with a success rate in obtaining saturation measurements varying between 20–100% at one minute after birth [18]. Several studies have found that reliable PO signals are rarely available in the first two minutes after birth [6–8,19,20]. A previous study by our team demonstrated that PO signal may be delayed in newborns with low APGAR scores, who represent the group in most need of HR feedback [7]. Others have evaluated the order of sensor application to the newborn with respect to the acquisition of a reliable PO signal [21–24], and video recordings in the present study showed that the practise did vary. The type of PO sensor used can also affect the time to a reliable signal during newborn resuscitations [25].

The results challenge the role of PO in the assessment of HR during newborn resuscitations. PO does, however, have an important role in the titration of oxygen provision during resuscitation in order to avoid hypoxia and hyperoxia with oxidative stress [25]. Although none of our videos showed a sign that PO disrupted or delayed PPV, the effort of placing PO rarely provided useful signal on HR or tissue oxygenation during ventilation.

Most resuscitations in our setting were of short duration with moderately asphyxiated newborns. PO may have a more prominent role in prolonged and advanced resuscitations or stabilization of preterms. PO is also used to confirm if the newborn has the capacity to maintain stable oxygenation within the recommended range [26], and may help identify newborns in need of admission to the neonatal intensive care unit.

Considerable resources went into the placement of PO. HCPs spent 30% of the time during active resuscitation applying PO, without obtaining PO signal in the majority of cases. Where resources are limited, prioritizing the placement of PO during ventilation may be impractical.

This study was limited by the loss of PO signal data in 104 newborns due to technical errors, including frame freezing of the monitor video and loss of resuscitation videos due to a server failure without a backup. In this study, we analysed the availability of PO signal during resuscitation, but have not evaluated the HR signal accuracy compared to the gold standard ECG. The population was limited to newborns with gestational age $\geq$28 weeks, since extremely premature newborns were resuscitated and stabilized in incubators not equipped with video cameras. The strengths of the study are the population-based design and a high number of included newborns. The setting is representative of high-resource contexts.

5. Conclusions

During delivery room resuscitation, 97% of newborns had PO applied in line with European Resuscitation Council Guideline recommendations. However, the application of PO was time-consuming, and PO signal were only displayed for 5% of the time of active resuscitation with PPV.

Author Contributions: Conceptualization, S.R., V.K., H.P. and H.E.; methodology, S.R., V.K., H.P., H.E. and J.E.; data extraction and processing, J.E. and V.K.; validation, S.R., V.K., H.P., H.E., J.E. and F.B.; formal analysis, S.R., V.K. and J.E.; investigation, V.K. and S.R.; resources, S.R. and H.E.; data curation, S.R., V.K., J.E. and F.B.; writing—original draft preparation, V.K. and S.R.; writing—review and editing, V.K., S.R., H.P., H.E., J.E. and F.B.; visualization, J.E., V.K. and F.B.; supervision, S.R. and H.E.; project administration, S.R.; funding acquisition, S.R. All authors have read and agreed to the published version of the manuscript.

Funding: This research was funded by Stavanger University Hospital and Laerdal Foundation (Safer Healthcare grant no 5007). The funders had no role in the design of the study; in the collection, analyses, or interpretation of data; in the writing of the manuscript; or in the decision to publish the results.

Institutional Review Board Statement: This study was conducted according to the guidelines of the Declaration of Helsinki and approved by the national Ethics Committee (reference number 2018/338), ethical date is 27 April 2018.

Informed Consent Statement: Informed consent was obtained from all subjects involved in the study.

Data Availability Statement: The data presented in this study are available on request from the corresponding author. The data are not publicly available due to privacy statements made in informed consent obtained from participants.

Acknowledgments: We thank participating mothers and their newborns, and HCPs at Stavanger University Hospital for taking part in the study.

Conflicts of Interest: J.E. is an employee at Laerdal Medical. S.R. received an unconditional research grant by Laerdal Foundation. The other four authors declare no conflict of interest.

References

1. Skare, C.; Kramer-Johansen, J.; Steen, T.; Odegaard, S.; Niles, D.E.; Nakstad, B.; Solevag, A.L.; Nadkarni, V.M.; Olasveengen, T.M. Incidence of Newborn Stabilization and Resuscitation Measures and Guideline Compliance during the First Minutes of Life in Norway. *Neonatology* **2015**, *108*, 100–107. [CrossRef] [PubMed]
2. Madar, J.; Roehr, C.C.; Ainsworth, S.; Ersdal, H.; Morley, C.; Rudiger, M.; Skare, C.; Szczapa, T.; Te Pas, A.; Trevisanuto, D.; et al. European Resuscitation Council Guidelines 2021: Newborn resuscitation and support of transition of infants at birth. *Resuscitation* **2021**, *161*, 291–326. [CrossRef] [PubMed]
3. Wyckoff, M.H.; Wyllie, J.; Aziz, K.; de Almeida, M.F.; Fabres, J.W.; Fawke, J.; Guinsburg, R.; Hosono, S.; Isayama, T.; Kapadia, V.S.; et al. Neonatal Life Support 2020 International Consensus on Cardiopulmonary Resuscitation and Emergency Cardiovascular Care Science With Treatment Recommendations. *Resuscitation* **2020**, *156*, A156–A187. [CrossRef] [PubMed]
4. Bjorland, P.A.; Oymar, K.; Ersdal, H.L.; Rettedal, S.I. Incidence of newborn resuscitative interventions at birth and short-term outcomes: A regional population-based study. *BMJ Paediatr. Open* **2019**, *3*, e000592. [CrossRef]
5. Wyckoff, M.H.; Greif, R.; Morley, P.T.; Ng, K.C.; Olasveengen, T.M.; Singletary, E.M.; Soar, J.; Cheng, A.; Drennan, I.R.; Liley, H.G.; et al. 2022 International Consensus on Cardiopulmonary Resuscitation and Emergency Cardiovascular Care Science with Treatment Recommendations: Summary from the Basic Life Support; Advanced Life Support; Pediatric Life Support; Neonatal Life Support; Education, Implementation, and Teams; and First Aid Task Forces. *Circulation* **2022**, *146*, e483–e557. [CrossRef]
6. Kamlin, C.O.; O'Donnell, C.P.; Everest, N.J.; Davis, P.G.; Morley, C.J. Accuracy of clinical assessment of infant heart rate in the delivery room. *Resuscitation* **2006**, *71*, 319–321. [CrossRef]
7. Bjorland, P.A.; Ersdal, H.L.; Oymar, K.; Rettedal, S.I. Compliance with guidelines and efficacy of heart rate monitoring during newborn resuscitation: A prospective video study. *Neonatology* **2020**, *117*, 175–181. [CrossRef]
8. Katheria, A.; Rich, W.; Finer, N. Electrocardiogram provides a continuous heart rate faster than oximetry during neonatal resuscitation. *Pediatrics* **2012**, *130*, e1177–e1181. [CrossRef]
9. Iglesias, B.; Rodriguez, M.J.; Aleo, E.; Criado, E.; Herranz, G.; Moro, M.; Martinez Orgado, J.; Arruza, L. Pulse oximetry versus electrocardiogram for heart rate assessment during resuscitation of the preterm infant. *Anales Pediatría* **2016**, *84*, 271–277. [CrossRef]
10. Mizumoto, H.; Tomotaki, S.; Shibata, H.; Ueda, K.; Akashi, R.; Uchio, H.; Hata, D. Electrocardiogram shows reliable heart rates much earlier than pulse oximetry during neonatal resuscitation. *Pediatr. Int.* **2012**, *54*, 205–207. [CrossRef]
11. Perlman, J.M.; Wyllie, J.; Kattwinkel, J.; Wyckoff, M.H.; Aziz, K.; Guinsburg, R.; Kim, H.S.; Liley, H.G.; Mildenhall, L.; Simon, W.M.; et al. Part 7: Neonatal resuscitation: 2015 international consensus on cardiopulmonary resuscitation and emergency cardiovascular care science with treatment recommendations. *Circulation* **2015**, *132* (Suppl. S1), S204–S241. [CrossRef]
12. van Vonderen, J.J.; Hooper, S.B.; Kroese, J.K.; Roest, A.A.; Narayen, I.C.; van Zwet, E.W.; te Pas, A.B. Pulse oximetry measures a lower heart rate at birth compared with electrocardiography. *J. Pediatr.* **2015**, *166*, 49–53. [CrossRef]
13. Johnson, P.A.; Cheung, P.Y.; Lee, T.F.; O'Reilly, M.; Schmolzer, G.M. Novel technologies for heart rate assessment during neonatal resuscitation at birth—A systematic review. *Resuscitation* **2019**, *143*, 196–207. [CrossRef]
14. Dawson, J.A.; Saraswat, A.; Simionato, L.; Thio, M.; Kamlin, C.O.; Owen, L.S.; Schmölzer, G.M.; Davis, P.G. Comparison of heart rate and oxygen saturation measurements from Masimo and Nellcor pulse oximeters in newly born term infants. *Acta Paediatr.* **2013**, *102*, 955–960. [CrossRef]
15. Rettedal, S.; Eilevstjonn, J.; Kibsgaard, A.; Kvaloy, J.T.; Ersdal, H. Comparison of Heart Rate Feedback from Dry-Electrode ECG, 3-Lead ECG, and Pulse Oximetry during Newborn Resuscitation. *Children* **2021**, *8*, 1092. [CrossRef]
16. Narayen, I.C.; Smit, M.; van Zwet, E.W.; Dawson, J.A.; Blom, N.A.; te Pas, A.B. Low signal quality pulse oximetry measurements in newborn infants are reliable for oxygen saturation but underestimate heart rate. *Acta Paediatr.* **2015**, *104*, e158–e163. [CrossRef]
17. Iglesias, B.; Rodri Guez, M.A.J.; Aleo, E.; Criado, E.; Marti Nez-Orgado, J.; Arruza, L. 3-lead electrocardiogram is more reliable than pulse oximetry to detect bradycardia during stabilisation at birth of very preterm infants. *Arch. Dis. Child. Fetal Neonatal Ed.* **2018**, *103*, F233–F237. [CrossRef]
18. Dawson, J.A.; Davis, P.G.; O'Donnell, C.P.; Kamlin, C.O.; Morley, C.J. Pulse oximetry for monitoring infants in the delivery room: A review. *Arch. Dis. Child. Fetal Neonatal Ed.* **2007**, *92*, F4–F7. [CrossRef]
19. Reddy, K.S.; Venkataravanappa, S.T.; Gururaja, G. Feasibility of Oxygen Saturation Monitoring During Neonatal Resuscitation in Indian Scenario. *Indian Pediatr.* **2018**, *55*, 999. [CrossRef]
20. Gandhi, B.; Rich, W.; Finer, N. Time to achieve stable pulse oximetry values in VLBW infants in the delivery room. *Resuscitation* **2013**, *84*, 970–973. [CrossRef]
21. Louis, D.; Sundaram, V.; Kumar, P. Pulse oximeter sensor application during neonatal resuscitation: A randomized controlled trial. *Pediatrics* **2014**, *133*, 476–482. [CrossRef] [PubMed]
22. O'Donnell, C.P.; Kamlin, C.O.; Davis, P.G.; Morley, C.J. Obtaining pulse oximetry data in neonates: A randomised crossover study of sensor application techniques. *Arch. Dis. Child. Fetal Neonatal Ed.* **2005**, *90*, F84–F85. [CrossRef] [PubMed]
23. Saraswat, A.; Simionato, L.; Dawson, J.A.; Thio, M.; Kamlin, C.O.; Owen, L.; Schmolzer, G.; Davis, P.G. Determining the best method of Nellcor pulse oximeter sensor application in neonates. *Acta Paediatr.* **2012**, *101*, 484–487. [CrossRef] [PubMed]
24. O'Donnell, C.P.; Kamlin, C.O.; Davis, P.G.; Morley, C.J. Feasibility of and delay in obtaining pulse oximetry during neonatal resuscitation. *J. Pediatr.* **2005**, *147*, 698–699. [CrossRef]

25. Baquero, H.; Alviz, R.; Castillo, A.; Neira, F.; Sola, A. Avoiding hyperoxemia during neonatal resuscitation: Time to response of different SpO2 monitors. *Acta Paediatr.* **2011**, *100*, 515–518. [CrossRef]
26. Boldingh, A.M.; Skare, C.; Nakstad, B.; Solevag, A.L. Suboptimal heart rate assessment and airway management in infants receiving delivery room chest compressions: A quality assurance project. *Arch. Dis. Child. Fetal Neonatal Ed.* **2020**, *105*, 545–549. [CrossRef]

children

MDPI

Article

The Genetics of Glucose-6-Phosphate-Dehydrogenase (G6PD) and Uridine Diphosphate Glucuronosyl Transferase 1A1 (UGT1A1) Promoter Gene Polymorphism in Relation to Quantitative Biochemical G6PD Activity Measurement and Neonatal Hyperbilirubinemia

Arieh Riskin [1,*], Yulia Bravdo [2], Clair Habib [2], Irit Maor [3], Julnar Mousa [4], Sizett Shahbarat [4], Elena Shahak [4] and Adel Shalata [4]

1 Department of Neonatology, Bnai Zion Medical Center, Ruth & Bruce Rappaport Faculty of Medicine, Technion, Israel Institute of Technology, Haifa 32000, Israel
2 Department of Pediatrics, Bnai Zion Medical Center, Ruth & Bruce Rappaport Faculty of Medicine, Technion, Israel Institute of Technology, Haifa 32000, Israel
3 Biochemistry Laboratory, Bnai Zion Medical Center, Ruth & Bruce Rappaport Faculty of Medicine, Technion, Israel Institute of Technology, Haifa 32000, Israel
4 The Simon Winter Institute for Human Genetics, Bnai Zion Medical Center, Ruth & Bruce Rappaport Faculty of Medicine, Technion, Israel Institute of Technology, Haifa 32000, Israel; adel.shalata@b-zion.org.il (A.S.)
* Correspondence: arik.riskin@gmail.com; Tel.: +972-50-6267330

Abstract: Glucose-6-phosphate dehydrogenase (G6PD) deficiency and polymorphism in uridine diphosphate glucuronosyl transferase 1A1 (UGT1A1) were associated with significant neonatal hyperbilirubinemia (NHB) and increased risk for kernicterus. However, quantitative screening tests for G6PD enzyme activity proved unsatisfactory in estimating the risk for significant NHB, especially in heterozygous females that could present phenotype overlap between normal homozygotes, heterozygotes, and deficient homozygotes, resulting in a continuum of intermediate G6PD activity. Objective: To examine the association of genotype and phenotype in newborns with decreased G6PD activity and its relation to NHB. Study design: Quantitative G6PD enzyme activities were measured on umbilical cord blood samples. After accepting parental consent, samples were analyzed for *G6PD* mutations and *UGT1A1* gene polymorphisms (number of TA repeats in the UGT1A1 promoter). The associations to quantitative G6PD activity and bilirubin levels were assessed. Results: 28 females and 27 males were studied. The *Mediterranean* mutation (*NM_001360016.2(G6PD): c.563C>T (p.Ser188Phe)*) was responsible for most cases of G6PD deficiency (20 hemizygous males, 3 homozygous and 16 heterozygous females). The association between this mutation, decreased G6PD activity and higher bilirubin levels was confirmed. Heterozygosity to 6/7 TA repeats in the *UGT1A1* promoter was associated with increased NHB, especially in female newborns with G6PD deficiency. However, it seems that the interaction between G6PD deficiency, *UGT1A1* promoter polymorphism, and NHB is more complex, possibly involving other genetic interactions, not yet described. Despite genotyping females with G6PD deficiency, the overlap between the upper range of borderline and the lower range of normal G6PD activity could not be resolved. Conclusions: The results of this study highlight the possibility for future implementation of molecular genetic screening to identify infants at risk for significant NHB, especially *UGT1A1* polymorphism in heterozygous females with borderline G6PD deficiency. However, further studies are needed before such screening could be applicable to daily practice.

Keywords: glucose-6-phosphate dehydrogenase (G6PD); uridine diphosphate glucuronosyl transferase 1A1 (UGT1A1); neonatal hyperbilirubinemia (NHB); genotype; phenotype; G6PD enzyme activity; G6PD deficiency; *Mediterranean* mutation; *UGT1A1* promoter polymorphism; number of TA repeats

1. Introduction

Neonatal hyperbilirubinemia (NHB) is a clinical condition frequently encountered in newborn infants. Careful evaluation and many times also management [1–3] are required, thus making NHB the most common reason for hospital readmission during the first week of life [4]. Although NHB is considered a benign transient physiological phenomenon in many neonates, in few infants total serum bilirubin (TSB) may rise to hazardous levels that pose a direct threat of an acute bilirubin encephalopathy that can lead to kernicterus and brain damage [5–12]. Genetic and environmental factors contribute to the development of NHB [1,2]. However, the important contribution of genetically determined conditions has been increasingly recognized in recent years [13–24]. Polymorphism across three genes was particularly reported in association with an increased risk for NHB including those of: (1) the red blood cell enzyme glucose-6-phosphate dehydrogenase (*G6PD*) [13,17,19–21,25–30]; (2) the hepatic bilirubin-conjugating enzyme uridine-diphosphate glucuronosyl transferase 1A1 (*UGT1A1*) [13,15–17,19,20,24,28,30–41]; and (3) the hepatic solute carrier organic anion transporter polypeptide 1B1 (*OATP1B1*)—the bilirubin transporter localized to the sinusoidal membrane of hepatocytes, which is the blood-hepatocyte interface that limits bilirubin hepatic uptake [18–20,42]. These genetic variants may interact with each other or with environmental contributors to produce significant NHB [19,20]. *UGT1A1* gene was investigated because of its significant role in bilirubin metabolism, namely hepatic bilirubin glucuronidation. The frequent polymorphism described in this gene was the insertion of a seventh (TA) repeat in the promoter sequence of *UGT1A1*, which usually consists of $(TA)_6$ repeats. The seventh (TA) repeat in the repetitive $(TA)_n$TAA element lessens the affinity of the TATAA binding protein, which is a transcription factor, to the TATAA box18, so that when the number of $(TA)_n$ repeats increase above the wild type $(TA)_6$, *UGT1A1* expression declines. The $(TA)_7/(TA)_7$ promoter homozygous variant has third of the wild-type UGT1A1 activity, and is responsible for Gilbert syndrome phenotype. Decreased hepatic bilirubin-conjugating capacity due to $(TA)_n$ promoter polymorphism was also associated with early-accelerated NHB and prolonged indirect hyperbilirubinemia, particularly in breastfed newborns. It can also increase the risk for significant NHB when coupled with hemolytic conditions. Co-expression of *UGT1A1* variants with other genes was frequently described. As many as two thirds of the individuals who were homozygous for the $(TA)_7$ *UGT1A1* promoter variant were also homozygous or heterozygous for the *OATP1B1* polymorphism. The co-expression *OATP1B1* polymorphism with *UGT1A1* variants could result in diminished hepatic bilirubin uptake with decreased hepatic bilirubin conjugation, impairing bilirubin clearance thus increasing hyperbilirubinemia. Many of the G6PD deficient individuals are homozygous or heterozygous to co-expression of the $(TA)_7$ variant on at least one allele. Co-expression of bilirubin conjugation-limiting gene variants seem to be important in modulating the risk for NHB, especially when coupled with other risk factors such as G6PD deficiency [19,20,29].

G6PD mutations are important contributors to the risk for significant NHB than can even lead to kernicterus [27]. *G6PD* gene variants may predispose to NHB by causing an acute hemolytic event with or without identifiable environmental trigger. Alternatively, *G6PD* mutations can lead to severe NHB by causing low-grade hemolysis coupled with *UGT1A1* gene polymorphisms [17,22,27–30,35]. *UGT1A1* promoter and coding sequence gene variants may cause significant NHB via decreased hepatic bilirubin conjugation [15–18,30–34,37–41].

Because G6PD deficiency is an X-linked condition, males may be either G6PD normal or deficient hemizygotes, whereas females may be either normal homozygotes, deficient homozygotes, or heterozygotes. Using biochemical testing, identification of the two male groups should be straightforward. Categorization of females, however, may be inaccurate. In any female cell, only one of the two X chromosomes is active. If the inactivation of the X chromosome was random, half of the cells of a heterozygote female would have been G6PD normal and half would have been deficient, and quantitative G6PD enzyme activity, representing both cell components, would have been intermediate between normal and deficient levels. However, X chromosome inactivation is usually nonrandom, resulting in varying proportions of red blood cells that may be either G6PD normal or deficient [43–45]. Thus, in heterozygous females, quantitative measurements of G6PD activities result in a continuum of borderline intermediate levels [46].

Immigration and inter-communal marriages spread G6PD deficiency beyond its original geographic and ethnic distribution. This should be taken into account when assessing risk factors for developing significant NHB. Israel is an immigrant country that absorbed Jews, including Sephardic Jews, coming from all over the world. Native Arabs and Jews originating from many countries comprise most of our population. Thus, our hospital has been one of the first in Israel to implement universal quantitative neonatal screening for G6PD deficiency in order to identify newborns at risk for developing severe NHB [47]. The ethnic characteristics of G6PD deficiency in our newborn population emphasized this approach [47]. A growing population of mixed ethnic origin (Ashkenazi and Sephardic Jewish intermarriages) was found, and 3.8% of the males in this group were G6PD deficient [47]. The World Health Organization (WHO) recommends screening all newborns in populations with a prevalence of 3 to 5% or more in males. Based on the data found on G6PD prevalence in our neonatal population, i.e., 4.5% of all males and even higher in some ethnic groups (10.7% in Sephardic Jews and 6.2% in Muslim Arabs) [47] our center, as well as other birthing medical centers in Israel, adopted a universal screening program for G6PD deficiency. Further justification for universal neonatal G6PD screening was the association between G6PD deficiency and significant NHB, including the increased risk associated with borderline intermediate G6PD activities in female infants [47]. However, the main pitfall of our current universal neonatal screening for G6PD deficiency is that it is a biochemical phenotype-based method. Quantitative measure of G6PD activity still lacks the genotypic equivalent that is so important for defining the infants, especially heterozygous female with intermediate G6PD activities, who may be at high risk for severe NHB and even kernicterus [27], not less than the deficient male infants. Using our universal screening data on quantitative measurements of G6PD activity in our entire population, the sex-based distribution of G6PD ranges of normal, deficient and intermediate activities was assessed [47]. However, the difficult challenge was to define the intermediate borderline range in female newborns. For clinical and practical considerations, adopting a reference value of G6PD activity <7 U/gHb for classifying male newborns as G6PD deficient was useful, although most *Mediterranean G6PD* deficient males in our population were with G6PD activities <2 U/gHb. However, it was hard to define the upper limit of G6PD activity for the intermediate continuum of borderline levels in the presumably heterozygous female groups. The suggested G6PD activity of 9.5 or 10 U/gHb for the upper limit [46,47] was the best approximation that could be achieved based on quantitative G6PD activity measurements without concomitant DNA analysis that was not readily available at that time.

Thus, the problem of identifying G6PD-deficient newborns at risk for significant NHB was not fully settled. Although most G6PD-deficient males can be accurately identified by quantitatively testing G6PD enzyme activity, females are more difficult to categorize because many in this group may be heterozygotes with phenotype overlap between normal homozygotes, heterozygotes, and deficient homozygotes [44]. Screening females by phenotypic biochemical quantitative enzymatic activity measurement is relatively inaccurate, and requires a wide range of safety zones in order not to miss any of these female infants at risk for severe NHB.

DNA-based polymerase chain reaction (PCR) molecular screening could probably be more accurate, because it identifies the exact genotype of these females. However this is usually more complicated and expensive technology, especially for setting up a screening program [44]. Another difficulty with DNA-based screening is the wide range of worldwide *G6PD* mutations [32,48,49]. Even if only considering the more frequent *G6PD* mutations in our region, dominated by $G6PD^{Mediterranean}$ that is common in Sephardic Jews and Arabs in our country, a significant number of mutations would still have to be screened for, because of the diverse population, being an immigration country [25,50–53].

The aim of this study was to examine another strategy to overcome the problem of defining the G6PD borderline deficiency range in relation to NHB. If our phenotypic biochemical quantitative G6PD enzymatic activity screening could be more accurate and reliable in identifying high-risk newborn infants, especially heterozygous females, then the need for genetic screening will decrease. Studying the specific possible genotypes associated with the different levels of G6PD activity in our population and their relations to the development and severity of NHB was thus the approach adopted. The goal of this study was to try to establish G6PD phenotype–genotype associations and relate them to the risk of developing severe NHB. This could be important in order to make our universal screening more clinically informative and practically efficient [44]. Specifically, the aim was to identify *G6PD* gene mutations in our population, identify *UGT1A1* promoter gene polymorphisms, and try to find the association with the biochemical G6PD activity and clinical NHB.

2. Materials and Methods

2.1. Study Population

Infants studied were born at the Bnai Zion medical center in Haifa. Based on the results of quantitative G6PD screening performed on all newborns in our hospital, male infants with G6PD deficiency (<7 U/gHb) and female infants with low and borderline G6PD levels (<12 U/gHb) were identified. The upper level of 12 U/gHb is beyond the upper limit of intermediate range (10 U/gHb) employed in clinical practice, because one of the study goals was to try and better define the upper limit of intermediate G6PD activity, and 12 U/gHb seemed to be a wide enough range to test. A small sample of male and female infants with normal G6PD activities (>7 U/gHb for males and >12 U/gHb for females) were included as controls.

2.2. Study Period

The period of the study was 1 August 2018–30 July 2021. Because of the COVID-19 pandemic with frequent lockdowns, and limited opportunities to obtain informed consents from both parents, sample collection was practically discontinued earlier than planned on 1 March 2020.

2.3. Consent

The parents of infants that qualified for genetic testing were approached by one of the first three authors (A.R., Y.B., and C.H.) for informed consent to use the same umbilical sample that was used for G6PD screening for further genetic analysis. All parents that were approached consented for the specific genetic analyses to be performed, as outlined below. However, this cannot be regarded as a cohort of all the infants with G6PD deficiency or borderline deficiency during the study period. Not all parents of infants that qualified for the study were approached because of different issues (i.e., weekends and holidays—if none of the authorized researchers was available to come and discuss consent with the parents; or pauses in collection of samples due to workload or technical issues in the involved laboratories).

2.4. Ethics

The study was approved by the local institutional review board (Helsinki committee) (0117-17-BNZ) on 23 July 2018 after also being approved by the supreme national review board of the Israeli Ministry of Health (Application number 044-2018) on 29 March 2018.

2.5. Measured Parameters

G6PD phenotype, i.e., G6PD activity, *G6PD* genotype, i.e., *G6PD* mutation (*Mediterranean* or other) and homozygosity or heterozygosity, *UGT1A1* gene polymorphisms, i.e., the number of TA repeats in the *UGT1A1* promoter, and bilirubin levels (either by non-invasive transcutaneous bilirubinometry or in serum from blood sample) were measured.

2.6. Study Design

Our suggested approach for studying G6PD genotype–phenotype relations and their association to NHB involved the following stages:

1. Developing a genetic methodology (high-resolution melting (HRM) analysis) that would enable us to easily identify mutant *G6PD* males and heterozygous and homozygous females compared to normal wild type *G6PD* controls.
2. Establishing a method to identify *UGT1A1* gene polymorphisms (number of TA repeats in the *UGT1A1* promoter) in normal and G6PD-deficient infants, and establish their associations with NHB in G6PD-deficient infants.
3. After establishing the method for identifying *G6PD* mutations in our population and their associations to specific *UGT1A1* gene polymorphisms associated with NHB, we checked the *G6PD* genotype in a sample of newborn infants, including females, who were allegedly heterozygotes. An infant's G6PD status was first identified by our universal umbilical cord blood's G6PD enzyme activity screening. For the purpose of this study, for female infants with intermediate G6PD activity measurements, the upper limit of intermediate range was widened beyond what is currently used (2–12 U/gHb). Before genetic testing, the parents of these infants were asked for their informed consent to use their infants' umbilical cord sample (taken in EDTA tube useful both for G6PD enzyme activity testing and for DNA mutation analysis) for genotype testing as part of this study.
4. Bilirubin levels of the infants studied were closely followed in order to identify whether they develop NHB and to define its severity. In this stage, our aim was to try to establish the phenotype–genotype relationships between the intermediate range of biochemically measured G6PD enzyme activity, the specific *G6PD* mutation, and the *UGT1A1* promoter gene polymorphisms that could identify infants, especially females, at risk for significant NHB.

2.7. Sample Size

For stages 1 and 2, recruitment of 50 infants was planned including infants with G6PD deficiency or borderline deficiency in a male: female ratio of 1:1, and ~15% infants with normal G6PD activity (>7 U/gHb for males (4) and >12 U/gHb for females (4)). For stage 3, recruitment of another 50 infants was planned: 10% males with G6PD deficiency (<7 U/gHb (5)) and 90% females with intermediate (2–12 U/gHb, higher upper level as discussed above) deficiency (45). As mentioned above, recruitment was discontinued on 1 March 2020 at the beginning of stage 3, before the desired sample size was reached. However, failure to establish HRM in our population as a fast low-cost method for identifying G6PD heterozygous and homozygous mutants without having to identify the exact mutation by sequencing also made efforts at continuation of recruitment to stage 3 after the end of the pandemic irrelevant.

2.8. Procedures

1. **Collection of blood samples for universal G6PD screening:** Universal screening for G6PD was implemented at the Bnai Zion Medical Center since July 2007 [47]. After delivery, umbilical cord blood samples for quantitative G6PD activity screening are routinely obtained. These are collected in ethylene diamine tetra acetic acid (EDTA) tubes that can also be used for DNA extraction and PCR analysis.
2. **Biochemical laboratory assays:**
   - 2.1 G6PD enzymatic activity was measured within two days of collection. Red cell G6PD activity was determined by the enzymatic colorimetric assay for quantitative determination of G6PD deficiency using a commercial kit (G6P-DH, Cat. No. 17.005, Sentinel Diagnostics, Milan, Italy). The quantitative test involves oxidation of glucose-6-phosphate to 6-phosphogluconate with concomitant reduction of NADP+ to NADPH. The rate of NADPH formation, which is proportional to G6PD activity, is measured spectrophotometrically.

The G6P-DH screening kit also contains Hemoglobin Normalization procedure, i.e., a rapid quantitative measurement of G6PD activity is coupled to a simultaneous evaluation of hemoglobin content. Results are expressed as units of activity per gram hemoglobin (U/gHb). All the tests of enzymatic activities were automatically run at 36 °C by the biochemistry analyzer, Cobas Mira (Roche diagnostic systems, Hoffman La-Roche LTD, Basel, Switzerland).

2.2 Total serum bilirubin (TSB) levels were spectrophotometrically determined by Twin Beam Analyzer (Gamidor Diagnostics Ltd., Petach Tikva, Israel,) at two wavelengths (455 nm and 575 nm).

3. **Transcutaneous bilirubinometry and clinical assessment of NHB:** Transcutaneous bilirubin (TcB) measurements were performed using the Minolta JM-105 (Dräger Jaundice meter—Biliblitz). TcB was measured routinely in all newborns at the time of discharge from the nursery (usually 52 ± 12 h after uncomplicated normal vaginal delivery). TSB was also measured if the TcB reading was higher than 11 mg/dL or the baby had known risk factors for significant neonatal hyperbilirubinemia. If both TcB and TSB were recorded, TSB was used for the analysis. Assessment of the severity of hyperbilirubinemia and decisions regarding phototherapy were based on the AAP guidelines [1] that were adopted by the Israeli Neonatal Association.
4. **Genetic laboratory analysis:** After obtaining parents' informed consent, DNA was extracted from the collected blood samples saved in EDTA tubes.

4.1 Complete PCR sequencing of the whole *G6PD* gene was performed, including the coding and the one non-coding exons, flanking intronic regions of the G6PD gene, and the *G6PD* gene 5′ and 3′ untranslated regions (5′UTR, 3′UTR). A list of the G6PD primers that were used can be found in the Supplementary Material section. In this method, one primer is used with dNTP and ddNTP nucleotides. ddNTP nucleotides are used as transmitters of the sequencing reaction. Because discontinuation of elongation is random, multiple fragments of DNA with different lengths are synthesized—each strand was stopped at a different point. A mixture of four ddNTP nucleotides, each carrying fluorophore with different fluorescent color, is used. At the stage of electrophoresis in the sequencer, the fluorescent signal is measured during the passage through the capillary in the optical cell. The information is electronically recorded, and the translated sequence is saved to the computer electronic database. Because this complete PCR sequencing is both time and cost consuming, initially it was planned only for a small number of representative samples—two of our control group were sequenced in order to verify a normal sequence. After that, the rest of the samples along with the control group were checked by GeneScan.

4.2 For all samples, employment of a new methodological approach to identify *G6PD* heterozygous and homozygous mutants using high resolution melting (HRM) analysis was planned. The advantage of using this method could be identification of *G6PD* heterozygous and homozygous mutants without identifying the exact mutation, as performed in sequencing, which should be faster and much less time and cost consuming. HRM is a new post-PCR analysis method used to identify genetic variation in nucleic acid sequences. It can discriminate DNA sequences based on their composition, length, GC content, or strand complementarity. HRM analysis starts with PCR amplification of the region of interest in the presence of a dsDNA-binding dye, which has high fluorescence when bound to dsDNA. The second step is a high-resolution melting step and capturing fluorescent data points per change in temperature. When the dsDNA dissociates into single strands, the dye is released which causes a change in fluorescence. Finally, a melt curve profile of the amplicon is received. Melt curves with similar shape but different melting temperature (Tm) represent homozygous variant samples compared to a wild type sample.

Melt curves with different shape are due to heterozygous variant samples. Tm is the point in the melt curve where 50% of the DNA is double-stranded and 50% is single-stranded (melted); it is visualized better in a first derivative curve (as a peak). After aligning the samples, the result is plotted and presented as the pre-melt region (100% fluorescence where every amplicon is double-stranded), active melt region (true fluorescence change), and post-melt region (0% fluorescence point where every amplicon is single-stranded). The differences between melt curves are often small and are best visualized using a difference plot that helps distinguish between the homozygous and heterozygous compared to the wild type. In order to detect unknown mutations, the whole gene was scanned. Using HRM analysis, scanning of the gene using 180 bp long amplicons with 25-mer forward and reverse primers and 25 bp overlap of each amplicon was initially done.

4.3 Initial HRM analysis of the first 10 male samples, although technically not optimal, compared with the melting curve of the normal *G6PD* sequence control group, revealed that the melting curve of exon 5 was different. Taking this into account and supported by published literature [54], exon 5 was directly sequenced and hemizygosity of the known *Mediterranean* mutation (*NM_001360016.2(G6PD): c.563C>T (p. Ser188Phe)*) was found in 6 out of 10 samples. Therefore, Sanger direct sequencing of exon 5 was the first step in all tested samples thereafter.

4.4 In order to find an association between the number of TA repeats (microsatellites) in the *UGT1A1* promoter and quantitative G6PD enzyme activity, especially in the heterozygous females, the number of TA repeats in the *UGT1A1* promoter was determined. Wild type *UGT1A1* contains six TA repeats [A(TA)$_6$TAA] in its promoter region [31]. Seven or more TA repeats was considered pathological. The analysis was performed using a sequencing method with primers that were specifically designed and synthesized for this purpose.

2.9. Statistical Analysis

Data were statistically analyzed using SigmaPlot, version 11.0 (Systat Software Inc. San Jose, CA, USA). Statistical analysis included descriptive statistics, and one-way analysis of variance (ANOVA) or chi-square test for comparisons of multiple continuous or categorical variables between groups. When appropriate, the non-parametric test of Kruskal–Wallis one-way analysis of variance on ranks was employed. Data are presented as mean ± standard deviation (SD) or median with interquartile range (IQR), as appropriate, and p-values of less than 0.05 are considered statistically significant.

3. Results

Fifty-five newborn infants were included in the study: 28 females and 27 males.

The *G6PD* gene has three different isoforms, as demonstrated in Figure 1, including 13 exons, and they differ in the first exon sequence, which is encoding only in *NM_000402.4(G6PD)* isoform.

According to the professional and public databases, there are 238 known damaging *G6PD* variants in the Human Gene Mutation Database (HGMD) and 299 pathogenic and 23 likely pathogenic variants in ClinVar (https://www.ncbi.nlm.nih.gov/clinvar, accessed on 12 June 2023). In our research group, the *NM_001360016.2(G6PD): c.563C>T (p.Ser188Phe)*, known as the *Mediterranean* pathogenic variant, was by far the most frequent mutation identified in our population, both in males and females. The *Mediterranean* pathogenic variant is also known as *NM_000402.4(G6PD):c.653C>T (p.Ser218Phe)* as explained in Figure 1 and illustrated at the genomic level in Figure 2 (30 codons shift (p.Ser188Phe p.Ser218Phe) due to exon 1 encoding only in isoform *NM_000402.4*).

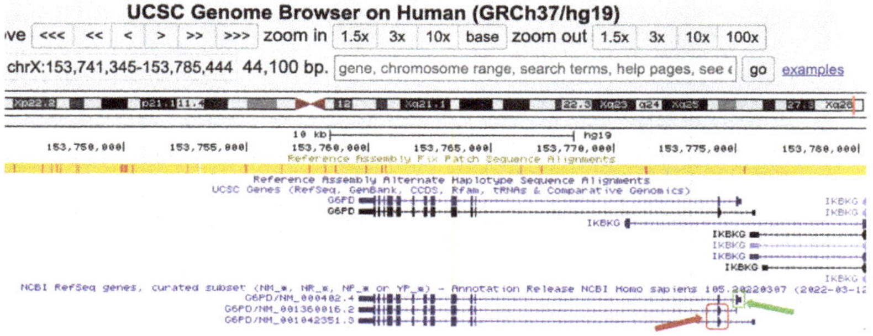

Figure 1. Screenshot of the *G6PD* different isoforms, *NM_000402.4*, *NM_001360016.2*, and *NM_1042351.3*, as illustrated in https://genome.ucsc.edu/, accessed on 12 June 2023. The *G6PD* isoforms differ in exon 1 where, exon 1 of NM_000402.4 is encoding (green arrow), while, in the other two isoforms exon 1 is not encoding. The first ATG start codon of both isoforms is located in the second exon (red rectangle). This fact can explain the difference in G6PD enzyme amino acid residue nomenclature in the *NM_000402.4* isoform compared to the *NM_001360016.2* and *NM_1042351.3* isoforms.

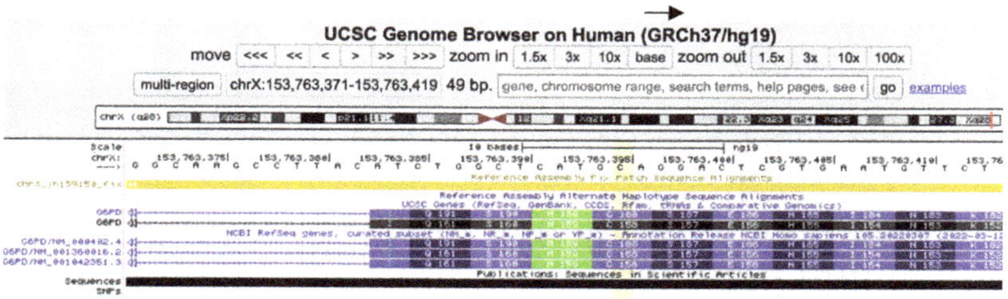

Figure 2. Screenshot of the Mediterranean *G6PD* mutation as demonstrated in https://genome.ucsc.edu/, accessed on 12 June 2023); the *NM_001360016.2(G6PD): c.563C>T (p. Ser188Phe)* (yellowish column) with its specific isoform nomenclature.

In the 27 male newborn infants' group, 20 males were hemizygous to the *Mediterranean* mutation (*NM_001360016.2(G6PD): c.563C>T (p. Ser188Phe)*) and seven did not have this mutation. All 20 hemizygous males with the *Mediterranean* mutation had very low G6PD activity of less than 1 U/gHb. The number of TA repeats in the *UGT1A1* promoter were 7/7 in three (abnormal homozygous), nine were heterozygous with 6/7 repeats, and eight were normal with 6/6 repeats. Among the seven males who were not found to have the *Mediterranean G6PD* deficiency mutation, three had G6PD activity lower than 7 U/gHb (in the range of 5–6.5). In this group of three, full sequencing of the *G6PD* gene was performed and other mutations of G6PD were found. Two of these infants were normal with 6/6 TA repeats in the *UGT1A1* promoter, and one was heterozygous with 6/7 repeats. The four other male infants without the *Mediterranean* or any other *G6PD* mutation had normal G6PD activity above 7 U/gHb. Three of these infants were normal with 6/6 TA repeats and one was heterozygous with 6/7 TA repeats in the *UGT1A1* promoter (Figure 3).

Of the 28 female newborn infants studied, three were homozygous to the *Mediterranean* mutation with low G6PD activity of 0–1.4 U/gHb in the biochemical quantitative assay. Genetically, two of these females were heterozygous with 6/7 TA repeats in the *UGT1A1* promoter, and the third was normal with 6/6 TA repeats (Figure 3).

Sixteen females were heterozygous to the *Mediterranean* mutation, 15 of them had no other *G6PD* mutation. Their G6PD activity was in the range of 6.2–11.6 U/gHb. Seven of this group had normal TA repeats (6/6) in the *UGT1A1* promoter, six were heterozygous with 6/7 repeats, and for the other two the blood sample was insufficient to complete this analysis and their data are missing. One female of the 16 *Mediterranean* heterozygous infants was also heterozygous to another *G6PD* mutation, defining her as compound heterozygous. Her G6PD activity was low—2 U/g Hb, and her genetic analysis revealed 6/7 TA repeats in the *UGT1A1* promoter (Figure 3).

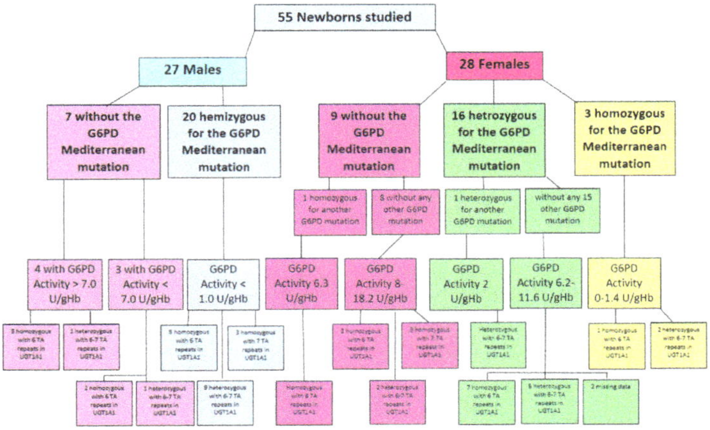

Figure 3. Study population by gender, *G6PD* mutation, G6PD activity, and number of TA repetitions in the *UGT1A1* promoter.

Nine of the 28 female infants did not have the *Mediterranean* mutation. Eight of them had no other *G6PD* deficiency mutation. Their G6PD activity in the biochemical assay was 8.8–18.2 U/gHb. Genetic analysis of the *UGT1A1* promoter revealed that three were homozygous with abnormal 7/7 TA repeats, two were heterozygous with 6/7 TA repeats and three were normal with 6/6 repeats. The last female in this group was homozygous for another *G6PD* mutation. Her G6PD activity was 6.3 U/gHb and UGT1A1 promoter analysis revealed 6/6 normal TA repeats (Figure 3).

Regarding G6PD activity, hemizygous male infants with the *Mediterranean* mutation had significantly lower G6PD activity. Although hemizygous males with another *G6PD* mutation demonstrated lower G6PD activity compared to males with normal G6PD activity, the difference was not statistically significant, most probably due to the relatively small group of such males in our sample (Table 1).

Homozygous and heterozygous G6PD-deficient females had lower G6PD activity compared to females without *G6PD* mutations. The homozygous females had low G6PD activities, and the heterozygous females had intermediate activities. The differences were statistically significant. Most of the *G6PD*-deficiency mutations were *Mediterranean*, as presented above. The few female infants with other *G6PD* mutations were subdivided for the analysis. The one who was compound heterozygous, i.e., heterozygous to two *G6PD* mutations, one of which was *Mediterranean*, was addressed as homozygous for G6PD deficiency. Another female who was homozygous to another (non-Mediterranean) *G6PD* mutation was analyzed with the female infants who were heterozygous to the *Mediterranean* mutation having intermediate G6PD activity (Table 1).

There was some overlap between the upper range of intermediate G6PD activity (6.2–11.6 U/gHb) in heterozygous female infants and lower range of normal G6PD activity (9.7–18.2 U/gHb) in female infants without mutations.

Although there were no significant differences in mean maximal bilirubin measured during nursery admission between the different genotypic *G6PD* groups of male and female newborns, there were some noteworthy differences (Table 1). Mean bilirubin level measured in the homozygous female infants was 9.3 mg/dL with levels that could reach as high as 20 mg/dL. Mean bilirubin level in the heterozygous females was slightly lower at 8.7 mg/dL with levels up to 18.5 mg/dL. In the group of females without *G6PD*

Mediterranean mutation, mean bilirubin level was lower at 7.4 mg/dL with a highest bilirubin level of 11.0 mg/dL measured in one of the infants (Table 1). Mean maximal bilirubin levels in the male infants were also not significantly different. In the group of 20 males who were hemizygous for the *Mediterranean* mutation, the highest bilirubin measured was 17.0 mg/dL as opposed to 12.2 mg/dL in the males with the normal *G6PD* genotype (Table 1).

Table 1. G6PD activity in male and female newborns by genetic profile and its association to maximal bilirubin levels measured in these infants.

Gender	n	*G6PD* Genotype	G6PD Activity (U/gHb)		*p*-Value	Maximal Bilirubin Level			*p*-Value
			Median	IQR		Median	IQR	Maximal Value	
Male	20	Hemizygous to the *Mediterranean G6PD* mutation	0.60 *	0.25–0.80	<0.001 *	9.35	7.45–11.85	17.0	0.138 ¶¶
	3	Hemizygous for another *G6PD* mutation	5.20	5.05–5.87		12.90	10.95–14.32	14.8	
	4	Normal	16.55 *	15.50–17.30		9.65	9.35–10.95	12.2	
Female	4	Homozygous **	1.00 †	0.30–1.70	<0.001 †¶	8.55	3.75–14.85	20.1	0.839 ¶¶
	16	Heterozygous ††	8.40 ¶	7.35–10.65		8.70	4.40–12.65	18.5	
	8	Normal	13.30 †¶	10.15–17.10		6.60	5.00–10.35	11.0	

IQR—Interquartile range (25–75% percentile). *—Kruskal–Wallis one-way analysis of variance on ranks (significantly different groups are marked by *). †—Kruskal–Wallis one-way analysis of variance on ranks (significantly different groups are marked by †). **—This group includes one female who was heterozygous for the Mediterranean mutation and also heterozygous for another G6PD mutation, i.e., compound heterozygous. ††—This group includes one female who was homozygous for another (non-Mediterranean) mutation. ¶—Kruskal–Wallis one-way analysis of variance on ranks (significantly different groups are marked by ¶). ¶¶—Kruskal–Wallis one-way analysis of variance on ranks.

Analyzing the number of TA repetitions in the UGT1A1 promoter revealed that the highest bilirubin levels were found in the two males hemizygous to the *Mediterranean* mutation who were also homozygous to 7/7 TA repeats (mean: 12.1 ± 0.3 mg/dL); and in the male who was hemizygous to another non-Mediterranean *G6PD* mutation who was heterozygous to 6/7 TA repeats (14.8 mg/dL). However, these were very small groups and the differences were not statistically significant (Table 2).

Table 2. G6PD genotype and UGT1A1 polymorphism in male and female newborns and their association to maximal bilirubin levels measured in these infants.

Gender	N	G6PD Genotype	UGT1A1 Promoter	n	Maximal Bilirubin Level		
			Number of TA Repeats		Median	IQR	*p*-Value
Male	20	Hemizygous to the Mediterranean G6PD mutation	6/6	9	9.50	7.82–12.30	0.199 *
			6/7	9	8.60	6.45–10.25	
			7/7	2	12.15	11.90–12.40	
	3	Hemizygous for another G6PD mutation	6/6	2	11.60	10.30–12.90	
			6/7	1	14.80	–	
	4	Normal	6/6	1	9.10	–	
			6/7	3	9.70	9.62–11.57	
Female	4	Homozygous **	6/6	1	7.50	–	0.698 *
			6/7	3	9.60	2.40–17.48	
	16	Heterozygous †	6/6	8	6.45	4.40–9.80	
			6/7	6	11.75	8.10–13.10	
			Unknown	2	8.60	3.70–13.50	
	8	Normal	6/6	3	5.60	5.52–8.82	
			6/7	2	10.90	10.80–11.00	
			7/7	3	4.50	4.20–6.82	

IQR—Interquartile range (25–75% percentile). *—Kruskal–Wallis one-way analysis of variance on ranks. **—This group includes one female who was heterozygous for the Mediterranean mutation and also heterozygous for another G6PD mutation, i.e., compound heterozygous. †—This group includes one female who was homozygous for another (non-Mediterranean) mutation.

In the females, heterozygosity to 6/7 TA repeats in the *UGT1A1* promoter was associated with the highest bilirubin levels (mean 10.1 ± 5.6 mg/dL, compared to 7.6 ± 4.1 in females with wild type *UGT1A1*, i.e., homozygous to 6/6 TA repeats in the promoter, and 5.4 ± 1.9 in homozygous with 7/7 TA repeats, p = 0.438) (Table 2).

Heterozygosity to 6/7 TA repeats in the UGT1A1 promoter in females was also associated with lower G6PD activity (mean 6.9 ± 4.0 U/gHb vs. 15.3 ± 4.1 in homozygous to 7/7 TA repeats and 9.5 ± 4.3 in homozygous to 6/6 TA repeats, p = 0.032).

4. Discussion

The *Mediterranean* pathogenic variant (*NM_001360016.2(G6PD): c.563C>T (p.Ser188Phe)*), also known as *NM_000402.4(G6PD):c.653C>T (p.Ser218Phe)* as explained in the results above (Figures 1 and 2), was associated in both hemizygous males and homozygous females with low G6PD activity. Heterozygous females with the *Mediterranean* mutation exhibited intermediate range G6PD activity with higher maximal bilirubin levels that were slightly lower than in the homozygous females with the mutation. Thus, the known association between the *Mediterranean G6PD* mutation and lower G6PD activity with higher levels of neonatal hyperbilirubinemia was confirmed [51].

Heterozygosity to 6/7 TA repeats in the promoter of *UGT1A1* was associated with more significant neonatal jaundice, especially if the newborn infant had complete or partial G6PD deficiency. This association seems to be more significant in females. However, from our analyses it seems that the interaction between G6PD deficiency and decreased conjugation by UGT1A1 because of incorrect number of TA repeats in the promoter with resultant increased neonatal hyperbilirubinemia without hemolysis [35] is more complex, and is possibly associated with other genetic interactions that have not yet been described [24].

However, it must be stressed that in this study only *UGT1A1* variants that had different polymorphisms in the promoter, and more specifically in the number of TA repeats in the $(TA)_n$TAA box of the promoter, were investigated [32,35,41]. The many other variants of the *UGT1A1* gene, which could significantly affect its activity and thus NHB, were not addressed [16,24,33]. Although Israel is an immigrant country with multiple diverse populations, many ethnic populations are under-represented or not represented in our population. There are many variants of *UGT1A1* and *G6PD* that have been described in the world [28,31,36–40] and were not addressed in this study; thus, their co-expression and effect on NHB deserve further studies in order to clarify the complex interactions that cause significant NHB.

Neonatal screening programs for G6PD increase parental and caretaker awareness, thereby facilitating early access to treatment with resultant diminished mortality and morbidity associated with severe NHB. Regarding our aim to try and better define the intermediate borderline G6PD activity range in females that are heterozygous to G6PD deficiency, so that these female infants could be better identified and their parents be guided before discharge from the nursery regarding the need for close follow-up for late-onset rapidly rising hyperbilirubinemia on days 4–6 of life, the genetic analysis was not helpful. Our results still demonstrate the overlap between the higher range of intermediate G6PD activity and the lower range of normal. Actually, in the range of 9.7–11.6 U/gHb there remains uncertainty that mandates caution in females with G6PD activity measured within this range. Thus, the threshold of normal G6PD activity in females, defined as 9.5 by Kaplan et al. [46,55] or 10 U/gHb by Riskin et al. [47], based on the distribution of G6PD activities measured by the biochemical method and the relation to NHB remains in doubt.

The main limitation of our study is our sample size that was affected by many factors including the costs of full genetic analysis. This was the result of our failure to establish HRM as a quick cheap method to identify *G6PD* mutations in our population instead of running full sequencing of the *G6PD* gene. This was quite surprising because HRM was successfully used in the past to identify *G6PD* mutations [56], including in our region [57]. Yet, it is possible that the combination of dominant *Mediterranean G6PD* mutation in our population along with the other *G6PD* mutations typical of our population as an immigrant country resulted in melting curves that were not sensitive enough to separate the mutations by HRM.

Regarding the possible contribution of analyzing the number of TA repeats in the *UGT1A1* promoter as another screening method to identify newborns, especially females, at risk for high NHB, it seems that the interaction with G6PD deficiency and significant neonatal jaundice is more complex, and requires further study and analysis before it can be recommended as a screening test for newborns. Recent studies highlight the independent role of the number of TA repeats in the *UGT1A1* promoter in NHB [24,38].

5. Conclusions

In summary, it is important to continue performing more studies to evaluate the role of genetic screening with analysis of the number of TA repeats in the *UGT1A1* promoter to assess for increased risk for NHB, especially in heterozygous females to G6PD deficiency. However, it cannot be recommended routinely at this time before more data and better interpretation of the genetic interactions are achieved.

Supplementary Materials: The following supporting information can be downloaded at: https://www.mdpi.com/article/10.3390/children10071172/s1, Table S1: G6PD primers that were used in this study.

Author Contributions: Conceptualization, A.R., Y.B., C.H. and A.S.; methodology, A.R., Y.B., C.H., I.M., J.M., S.S., E.S. and A.S.; software, J.M., S.S., E.S. and A.S.; validation, J.M., S.S., E.S. and A.S.; formal analysis, A.R., J.M., S.S., E.S. and A.S.; investigation, A.R., Y.B., J.M., S.S., E.S. and A.S.; resources, A.R. and A.S.; data curation, Y.B. and C.H.; writing—original draft preparation, A.R.; writing—review and editing, Y.B., C.H., I.M., J.M., S.S., E.S. and A.S.; supervision, A.R., I.M. and A.S.; funding acquisition, A.R. All authors have read and agreed to the published version of the manuscript.

Funding: This research was funded by the ALBERT GOODSTEIN RESEARCH FUND, grant number 2025088, Executive Vice President of Research Office, Israel Institute of Technology, Ref. A/1015451, 17 September 2017.

Institutional Review Board Statement: The study was approved by the local institutional review board (Helsinki committee) (0117-17-BNZ) on 23 July 2018 after being approved also by the supreme national review board of the Israeli Ministry of Health (Application number 044-2018) on 29 March 2018.

Informed Consent Statement: Informed consent was obtained from all parents of the newborns involved in the study.

Data Availability Statement: Data is unavailable due to privacy and ethical restrictions as dictated by the Helsinki committees.

Conflicts of Interest: The authors declare no conflict of interest. The funders had no role in the design of the study; in the collection, analyses, or interpretation of data; in the writing of the manuscript; or in the decision to publish the results.

References

1. American Academy of Pediatrics Subcommittee on Hyperbilirubinemia. Management of hyperbilirubinemia in the newborn infant 35 or more weeks of gestation. *Pediatrics* **2004**, *114*, 297–316. [CrossRef] [PubMed]
2. Kemper, A.R.; Newman, T.B.; Slaughter, J.L.; Maisels, M.J.; Watchko, J.F.; Downs, S.M.; Grout, R.W.; Bundy, D.G.; Stark, A.R.; Bogen, D.L.; et al. Clinical Practice Guideline Revision: Management of Hyperbilirubinemia in the Newborn Infant 35 or More Weeks of Gestation. *Pediatrics* **2022**, *150*, e2022058859. [CrossRef] [PubMed]
3. Slaughter, J.L.; Kemper, A.R.; Newman, T.B. Technical Report: Diagnosis and Management of Hyperbilirubinemia in the Newborn Infant 35 or More Weeks of Gestation. *Pediatrics* **2022**, *150*, e2022058865. [CrossRef] [PubMed]
4. Maisels, M.J.; Kring, E. Length of stay, jaundice, and hospital readmission. *Pediatrics* **1998**, *101*, 995–998. [CrossRef] [PubMed]
5. Bhutani, V.K.; Johnson, L.H. Newborn jaundice and kernicterus—Health and societal perspectives. *Indian J. Pediatr.* **2003**, *70*, 407–416. [CrossRef] [PubMed]
6. Newman, T.B.; Maisels, M.J. How to avoid kernicterus. *J. Pediatr.* **2003**, *142*, 212–213, author reply 214–215. [CrossRef]
7. Bhutani, V.K.; Donn, S.M.; Johnson, L.H. Risk management of severe neonatal hyperbilirubinemia to prevent kernicterus. *Clin. Perinatol.* **2005**, *32*, 125–139. [CrossRef] [PubMed]
8. Bhutani, V.K. Kernicterus as a 'Never-Event': A newborn safety standard? *Indian J. Pediatr.* **2005**, *72*, 53–56. [CrossRef]
9. Bhutani, V.K.; Johnson, L. Kernicterus in the 21st century: Frequently asked questions. *J. Perinatol.* **2009**, *29* (Suppl. S1), S20–S24. [CrossRef]
10. Bhutani, V.K.; Johnson, L. A proposal to prevent severe neonatal hyperbilirubinemia and kernicterus. *J. Perinatol.* **2009**, *29* (Suppl. S1), S61–S67. [CrossRef] [PubMed]
11. Stevenson, D.K.; Wong, R.J.; Vreman, H.J.; McDonagh, A.F.; Maisels, M.J.; Lightner, D.A. NICHD Conference on Kernicterus: Research on Prevention of Bilirubin-Induced Brain Injury and Kernicterus: Bench-to-Bedside—Diagnostic Methods and Prevention and Treatment Strategies. *J. Perinatol.* **2004**, *24*, 521–525. [CrossRef] [PubMed]
12. Maisels, M.J. Neonatal hyperbilirubinemia and kernicterus—Not gone but sometimes forgotten. *Early Human Dev.* **2009**, *85*, 727–732. [CrossRef]
13. Kaplan, M.; Hammerman, C. Bilirubin and the genome: The hereditary basis of unconjugated neonatal hyperbilirubinemia. *Curr. Pharmacogenomics* **2005**, *3*, 21–42. [CrossRef]
14. Watchko, J.F.; Daood, M.J.; Biniwale, M. Understanding neonatal hyperbilirubinaemia in the era of genomics. *Semin. Neonatol. SN* **2002**, *7*, 143–152. [CrossRef] [PubMed]
15. Bosma, P.J. Inherited disorders of bilirubin metabolism. *J. Hepatol.* **2003**, *38*, 107–117. [CrossRef] [PubMed]
16. Kadakol, A.; Ghosh, S.S.; Sappal, B.S.; Sharma, G.; Chowdhury, J.R.; Chowdhury, N.R. Genetic lesions of bilirubin uridine-diphosphoglucuronate glucuronosyltransferase (UGT1A1) causing Crigler-Najjar and Gilbert syndromes: Correlation of genotype to phenotype. *Hum. Mutat.* **2000**, *16*, 297–306. [CrossRef]
17. Kaplan, M.; Renbaum, P.; Levy-Lahad, E.; Hammerman, C.; Lahad, A.; Beutler, E. Gilbert syndrome and glucose-6-phosphate dehydrogenase deficiency: A dose-dependent genetic interaction crucial to neonatal hyperbilirubinemia. *Proc. Natl. Acad. Sci. USA* **1997**, *94*, 12128–12132. [CrossRef]
18. Huang, M.J.; Kua, K.E.; Teng, H.C.; Tang, K.S.; Weng, H.W.; Huang, C.S. Risk factors for severe hyperbilirubinemia in neonates. *Pediatr. Res.* **2004**, *56*, 682–689. [CrossRef]
19. Lin, Z.; Fontaine, J.; Watchko, J.F. Coexpression of gene polymorphisms involved in bilirubin production and metabolism. *Pediatrics* **2008**, *122*, e156–e162. [CrossRef]
20. Watchko, J.F.; Lin, Z. Exploring the genetic architecture of neonatal hyperbilirubinemia. *Semin. Fetal Neonatal Med.* **2010**, *15*, 169–175. [CrossRef]
21. Mason, P.J.; Bautista, J.M.; Gilsanz, F. G6PD deficiency: The genotype-phenotype association. *Blood Rev.* **2007**, *21*, 267–283. [CrossRef] [PubMed]
22. Watchko, J.F.; Lin, Z.; Clark, R.H.; Kelleher, A.S.; Walker, M.W.; Spitzer, A.R.; Pediatrix Hyperbilirubinemia Study Group. Complex multifactorial nature of significant hyperbilirubinemia in neonates. *Pediatrics* **2009**, *124*, e868–e877. [CrossRef] [PubMed]
23. Kaplan, M.; Hammerman, C.; Maisels, M.J. Bilirubin genetics for the nongeneticist: Hereditary defects of neonatal bilirubin conjugation. *Pediatrics* **2003**, *111*, 886–893. [CrossRef]

24. Watchko, J.F. The contribution of genetic factors to hyperbilirubinemia and kernicterus risk in neonates: A targeted update. *Pediatr. Med.* **2021**, *4*, 17. [CrossRef]
25. Cappellini, M.D.; Fiorelli, G. Glucose-6-phosphate dehydrogenase deficiency. *Lancet* **2008**, *371*, 64–74. [CrossRef]
26. Arain, Y.H.; Bhutani, V.K. Prevention of Kernicterus in South Asia: Role of neonatal G6PD deficiency and its identification. *Indian J. Pediatr.* **2014**, *81*, 599–607. [CrossRef]
27. Kaplan, M.; Hammerman, C. Glucose-6-phosphate dehydrogenase deficiency: A hidden risk for kernicterus. *Semin. Perinatol.* **2004**, *28*, 356–364. [CrossRef]
28. Chavez-Pena, T.; Martinez-Camberos, A.; Cossio-Gurrola, G.; Arambula-Meraz, E.; Herrera-Rodriguez, I.; Romo-Martinez, E.; Garcia-Magallanes, N. Prevalence of UGT1A1 (TA)n promoter polymorphism in Panamanians neonates with G6PD deficiency. *J. Genet.* **2020**, *99*, 63. [CrossRef]
29. Kaplan, M.; Hammerman, C. Glucose-6-phosphate dehydrogenase deficiency and severe neonatal hyperbilirubinemia: A complexity of interactions between genes and environment. *Semin. Fetal Neonatal Med.* **2010**, *15*, 148–156. [CrossRef]
30. Huang, C.S.; Chang, P.F.; Huang, M.J.; Chen, E.S.; Chen, W.C. Glucose-6-phosphate dehydrogenase deficiency, the UDP-glucuronosyl transferase 1A1 gene, and neonatal hyperbilirubinemia. *Gastroenterology* **2002**, *123*, 127–133. [CrossRef]
31. Vukovic, M.; Radlovic, N.; Lekovic, Z.; Vucicevic, K.; Maric, N.; Kotur, N.; Gasic, V.; Ugrin, M.; Stojiljkovic, M.; Dokmanovic, L.; et al. UGT1A1 (TA)(n) Promoter Genotype: Diagnostic and Population Pharmacogenetic Marker in Serbia. *Balk. J. Med. Genet. BJMG* **2018**, *21*, 59–68. [CrossRef] [PubMed]
32. Muslu, N.; Turhan, A.B.; Eskandari, G.; Atici, A.; Ozturk, O.G.; Kul, S.; Atik, U. The frequency of UDP-glucuronosyltransferase 1A1 promoter region (TA)7 polymorphism in newborns and it's relation with jaundice. *J. Trop. Pediatr.* **2007**, *53*, 64–68. [CrossRef] [PubMed]
33. Hanchard, N.A.; Skierka, J.; Weaver, A.; Karon, B.S.; Matern, D.; Cook, W.; O'Kane, D.J. UGT1A1 sequence variants and bilirubin levels in early postnatal life: A quantitative approach. *BMC Med. Genet.* **2011**, *12*, 57. [CrossRef] [PubMed]
34. Pasha, Y.Z.; Kacho, M.A.; Niaki, H.A.; Tarighati, M.; Alaee, E. The association between prolonged jaundice and TATA box dinucleotide repeats in Gilbert's syndrome. *J. Clin. Diagn. Res.* **2017**, *11*, GC05–GC07. [CrossRef]
35. Kaplan, M.; Renbaum, P.; Vreman, H.J.; Wong, R.J.; Levy-Lahad, E.; Hammerman, C.; Stevenson, D.K. (TA)n UGT 1A1 promoter polymorphism: A crucial factor in the pathophysiology of jaundice in G-6-PD deficient neonates. *Pediatr. Res.* **2007**, *61*, 727–731. [CrossRef]
36. Babaoglu, M.O.; Yigit, S.; Aynacioglu, A.S.; Kerb, R.; Yurdakok, M.; Bozkurt, A. Neonatal jaundice and bilirubin UDP-glucuronosyl transferase 1A1 gene polymorphism in Turkish patients. *Basic Clin. Pharmacol. Toxicol.* **2006**, *98*, 377–380. [CrossRef]
37. Amandito, R.; Rohsiswatmo, R.; Carolina, E.; Maulida, R.; Kresnawati, W.; Malik, A. Profiling of UGT1A1*6, UGT1A1*60, UGT1A1*93, and UGT1A1*28 Polymorphisms in Indonesian Neonates with Hyperbilirubinemia Using Multiplex PCR Sequencing. *Front. Pediatr.* **2019**, *7*, 328. [CrossRef]
38. Yang, H.; Wang, Q.; Zheng, L.; Zheng, X.B.; Lin, M.; Zhan, X.F.; Yang, L.Y. Clinical Significance of UGT1A1 Genetic Analysis in Chinese Neonates with Severe Hyperbilirubinemia. *Pediatr. Neonatol.* **2016**, *57*, 310–317. [CrossRef]
39. Agrawal, S.K.; Kumar, P.; Rathi, R.; Sharma, N.; Das, R.; Prasad, R.; Narang, A. UGT1A1 gene polymorphisms in North Indian neonates presenting with unconjugated hyperbilirubinemia. *Pediatr. Res.* **2009**, *65*, 675–680. [CrossRef]
40. Beutler, E.; Gelbart, T.; Demina, A. Racial variability in the UDP-glucuronosyltransferase 1 (UGT1A1) promoter: A balanced polymorphism for regulation of bilirubin metabolism? *Proc. Natl. Acad. Sci. USA* **1998**, *95*, 8170–8174. [CrossRef]
41. Kringen, M.K.; Piehler, A.P.; Grimholt, R.M.; Opdal, M.S.; Haug, K.B.; Urdal, P. Serum bilirubin concentration in healthy adult North-Europeans is strictly controlled by the UGT1A1 TA-repeat variants. *PLoS ONE* **2014**, *9*, e90248. [CrossRef] [PubMed]
42. Watchko, J.F. Genetics and the risk of neonatal hyperbilirubinemia: Commentary on the article by Huang et al. on page 682. *Pediatr. Res.* **2004**, *56*, 677–678. [CrossRef] [PubMed]
43. Kaplan, M.; Beutler, E.; Vreman, H.J.; Hammerman, C.; Levy-Lahad, E.; Renbaum, P.; Stevenson, D.K. Neonatal hyperbilirubinemia in glucose-6-phosphate dehydrogenase-deficient heterozygotes. *Pediatrics* **1999**, *104*, 68–74. [CrossRef]
44. Kaplan, M.; Hammerman, C. Neonatal screening for glucose-6-phosphate dehydrogenase deficiency: Biochemical versus genetic technologies. *Semin. Perinatol.* **2011**, *35*, 155–161. [CrossRef] [PubMed]
45. Lyon, M.F. X-chromosome inactivation and human genetic disease. *Acta Paediatr.* **2002**, *91*, 107–112. [CrossRef]
46. Algur, N.; Avraham, I.; Hammerman, C.; Kaplan, M. Quantitative neonatal glucose-6-phosphate dehydrogenase screening: Distribution, reference values, and classification by phenotype. *J. Pediatr.* **2012**, *161*, 197–200. [CrossRef] [PubMed]
47. Riskin, A.; Gery, N.; Kugelman, A.; Hemo, M.; Spevak, I.; Bader, D. Glucose-6-phosphate dehydrogenase deficiency and borderline deficiency: Association with neonatal hyperbilirubinemia. *J. Pediatr.* **2012**, *161*, 191–196.e191. [CrossRef]
48. Gomez-Manzo, S.; Marcial-Quino, J.; Vanoye-Carlo, A.; Serrano-Posada, H.; Ortega-Cuellar, D.; Gonzalez-Valdez, A.; Castillo-Rodriguez, R.A.; Hernandez-Ochoa, B.; Sierra-Palacios, E.; Rodriguez-Bustamante, E.; et al. Glucose-6-Phosphate Dehydrogenase: Update and Analysis of New Mutations around the World. *Int. J. Mol. Sci.* **2016**, *17*, 2069. [CrossRef]
49. Geck, R.C.; Powell, N.R.; Dunham, M.J. Functional interpretation, cataloging, and analysis of 1,341 glucose-6-phosphate dehydrogenase variants. *Am. J. Hum. Genet.* **2023**, *110*, 228–239. [CrossRef]
50. Kurdi-Haidar, B.; Mason, P.J.; Berrebi, A.; Ankra-Badu, G.; al-Ali, A.; Oppenheim, A.; Luzzatto, L. Origin and spread of the glucose-6-phosphate dehydrogenase variant (G6PD-Mediterranean) in the Middle East. *Am. J. Hum. Genet.* **1990**, *47*, 1013–1019.

51. Oppenheim, A.; Jury, C.L.; Rund, D.; Vulliamy, T.J.; Luzzatto, L. G6PD Mediterranean accounts for the high prevalence of G6PD deficiency in Kurdish Jews. *Human Genet.* **1993**, *91*, 293–294. [CrossRef] [PubMed]
52. Sirdah, M.; Reading, N.S.; Vankayalapati, H.; Perkins, S.L.; Shubair, M.E.; Aboud, L.; Roper, D.; Prchal, J.T. Molecular heterogeneity of glucose-6-phosphate dehydrogenase deficiency in Gaza Strip Palestinians. *Blood Cells Mol. Dis.* **2012**, *49*, 152–158. [CrossRef] [PubMed]
53. Abu Omar, R.; Algur, N.; Megged, O.; Hammerman, C.; Kaplan, M. Glucose-6-Phosphate Dehydrogenase Screening in Israel-Arab and Palestinian-Arab Neonates. *J. Pediatr.* **2015**, *167*, 169–172. [CrossRef]
54. Calabro, V.; Giacobbe, A.; Vallone, D.; Montanaro, V.; Cascone, A.; Filosa, S.; Battistuzzi, G. Genetic heterogeneity at the glucose-6-phosphate dehydrogenase locus in southern Italy: A study on a population from the Matera district. *Human Genet.* **1990**, *86*, 49–53. [CrossRef] [PubMed]
55. Kaplan, M.; Algur, N.; Hammerman, C. Intermediate values of glucose-6-phosphate dehydrogenase. *J. Pediatr.* **2012**, *161*, 571. [CrossRef]
56. Yan, J.B.; Xu, H.P.; Xiong, C.; Ren, Z.R.; Tian, G.L.; Zeng, F.; Huang, S.Z. Rapid and reliable detection of glucose-6-phosphate dehydrogenase (G6PD) gene mutations in Han Chinese using high-resolution melting analysis. *J. Mol. Diagn. JMD* **2010**, *12*, 305–311. [CrossRef] [PubMed]
57. Joly, P.; Lacan, P.; Garcia, C.; Martin, C.; Francina, A. Rapid genotyping of two common G6PD variants, African (A-) and Mediterranean, by high-resolution melting analysis. *Clin. Biochem.* **2010**, *43*, 193–197. [CrossRef]

children

MDPI

Article

Cerebral Myelination in a Bronchopulmonary Dysplasia Murine Model

Wenwen Chen [1,2,3], Ran Wang [1,2] and Chao Chen [1,2,*]

1 Children's Hospital of Fudan University, Shanghai 201102, China; pipixiu@163.com (W.C.); 20111240016@fudan.edu.cn (R.W.)
2 Key Laboratory of Neonatal Diseases, National Health Commission, Shanghai 201102, China
3 Zhangzhou Municipal Hospital of Fujian Province, Zhangzhou 363000, China
* Correspondence: chaochen@fudan.edu.cn or chen6010@163.com

Abstract: Introduction: Bronchopulmonary dysplasia (BPD) is a devastating disease in preterm infants concurrent with neurodevelopmental disorders. Chronic hyperoxia exposure might also cause brain injury, but the evidence was insufficient. Methods: Neonatal C57BL/6J mice were exposed to hyperoxia from P0 to induce a BPD disease model. Lung histopathological morphology analyses were performed at P10, P15, and P20. Cerebral myelination was assessed using MBP (myelin basic protein, a major myelin protein), NfH (neurofilament heavy chain, a biomarker of neurofilament heavy chain), and GFAP (glial fibrillary acidic protein, a marker of astrocytes) as biomarkers by western blot and immunofluorescence. Results: Mice exposed to hyperoxia exhibited reduced and enlarged alveoli in lungs. During hyperoxia exposure, MBP declined at P10, but then increased to a comparable level to the air group at P15 and P20. Meanwhile, GFAP elevated significantly at P10, and the elevation sustained to P15 and P20. Conclusion: Neonatal hyperoxia exposure caused an arrest of lung development, as well as an obstacle of myelination process in white matter of the immature brain, with a decline of MBP in the generation period of myelin and persistent astrogliosis.

Keywords: neonatal hyperoxia; molecular injury; cerebral myelination

1. Introduction

Neonatal hyperoxia exposure is frequent among preterm infants for lifesaving, particularly among those born with respiratory distress before 32 weeks of gestational age. For infants born preterm, even breathing the room's normal air is hyperoxia relative to the fetus' environment. Hyperoxia adds oxidative stress to the process of subsequent organ development after birth that might lead to developmental disturbances. Notably, hyperoxia is considered to be the key contributor to bronchopulmonary dysplasia (BPD). BPD seems to be a predictor of functional, behavioral, and sensory deficits [1]. As shown by the literature, lower cognitive scores assessed by Bayley III were more common in preterm-born children with BPD at 18–24 months of corrected age [2]. However, the mechanism underlying neurodevelopmental disturbances in BPD infants are not completely understood.

Encephalopathy of prematurity (EoP) is a major pattern of brain injury in preterm infants, characterized by widespread hypomyelination or diffuse white matter injury (WMI). It is generally accepted that EoP is caused by systemic perinatal inflammation from infection and/or hypoxia-ischemia, with strong evidence revealed by animal models that mimic perinatal conditions [3,4]. Recently, hyperoxia-induced brain injury has attracted attention, since it represents a realistic clinical insult that preterm infants encounter during the transitional period at birth. Several experimental studies demonstrated that hyperoxia damaged mitochondrial function in the brain [5], induced oligodendrocytes degeneration [6], and generated long-term cognitive deficits [7]. During normal human brain development, the formation of myelin sheaths by oligodendrocytes spurts a rapid brain growth that is known as cerebral myelination, at around 30 weeks of gestational age until two years of age, whereas the growth spurt of myelin in rodents is around postnatal day 2 (P2) to P10 [8]. Thus, infants born during this key period are vulnerable to brain injuries. Whether BPD-associated brain injury is caused by intermittent or continuous hypoxia owing to deteriorative lung function or attributed to direct hyperoxia injury is controversial. Direct evidence of negative effects that hyperoxia imposes on the process of myelination is still lacking.

In view of this, we addressed the impact of neonatal hyperoxia on the process of myelination in the same experimental model as BPD, with the aim to reveal the molecular substratum of hyperoxia-associated brain injury from a dynamic perspective.

2. Methods

2.1. Animals and Hyperoxia Intervention

C57BL/6 J mice were purchased from JieSiJie Laboratory Animal Co., Ltd., Shanghai, China, and were housed in animal care facilities at Fudan University Affiliated Pudong Medical Center, Shanghai, China (approval code: XYXKHU2020-0005). Animal procedures were performed in accordance with the Institutional Animal Care and Use Committee (IACUC) of Fudan University (approval code: 00033).

The female adult mice mated 3:1 with the male in the afternoon and were separated the next morning. To establish hyperoxia-induced models, newborn pups were exposed to 80% hyperoxia at birth (postnatal day 0, P0) along with their mothers, in cages in an airtight Plexiglass chamber (size 80 cm × 35 cm × 30 cm with two holes on the side walls for inputting oxygen and air escape) with a continuous import of oxygen (1 L/min). The fraction of inspiration oxygen was measured by an oxygen analyzer to maintain 80% in the hyperoxia group. This method and oxygen concentration were adopted generally by researchers to stably establish an experimental BPD phenotype [9]. Animals were raised at 22~27 °C with 50~70% humidity and subjected to a 12 h light–dark cycle. Soda lime was used to absorb CO_2, and silica gel beads were used to absorb H_2O. Hyperoxia exposure lasted 10 days, 15 days, and 20 days, respectively, and pups were sacrificed at corresponding time points at P10, P15, and P20 for lung and brain harvest. Age-matched control mice were housed in normal room air. Pups were kept with their mothers from the start to the end in the hyperoxia environment, and mothers were exchanged between air and hyperoxia groups every 24 h to avoid oxygen toxicity. Mice were grouped by block randomization. At the time of tissue harvest, mice were euthanized by 5% isoflurane inhalation. The chest cavity was exposed, the left auricle was cut, and the lungs were cleared of blood by perfusion with cold PBS via the right ventricle. The lungs were inflated with 4% paraformaldehyde under constant pressure of 30 cm water until the edges swelled and allowed to fix in 4% paraformaldehyde for 24 h for further paraffin section following dehydration. The brains were removed with careful elimination of the olfactory bulb after a scission at the back of the neck, posterior median line, and skull. A portion of the brain tissues were fixed in 4% paraformaldehyde for further freezing, and the others were stored in a −80 °C refrigerator after quick freezing in liquid nitrogen for further western blot analyses.

2.2. Hematoxylin-Eosin (HE) Staining and Lung Morphological Assessment

HE staining is a convenient and effective method to show cellular morphology and lung structure, providing a merit for recognizing some pathological patterns and parameter measurements. It is generally accepted for pathological diagnosis and morphological assessment of BPD phenotype in research. The fixed lungs were embedded with paraffin after gradient dehydration with a series of ethanol and xylene, and then cut into 3.5-μm-thick sections. Three tissue sections of each pup were selected for analysis. The sections were dewaxed, hydrated, and stained with hematoxylin and eosin. After staining, sections were dehydrated through increasing concentrations of ethanol and xylene, and then observed under an optical microscope. Images were taken at 40 multiplying power by an image acquisition system. Then images were observed on computer by K-Viewer software, and lung morphological analysis was performed on ten fields of each section manually. Radial alveolar count (RAC), representing alveologenesis [10], and mean linear intercept (MLI) [11]—representing the average alveolar diameter—were used for pulmonary morphological parameters. RAC counts were performed by magnifying by 4 times, superimposing the primary images. A perpendicular was dropped from the center of a bronchiole to the edge of the acinus (connective tissue septum or pleura), and the number of alveoli cut by this line was counted. MLI (Lm) calculations were done by magnifying by 10 times, superimposing the primary images. A grid was superimposed over each image, and the number of times the alveolar walls intercepted the grid lines was counted. The equation $Lm = (N)(L)/m$, where N = number of times the transverses were placed on the tissue, L = length of the transverses, and m = the sum of all intercepts, gave Lm.

2.3. Immunofluorescence of Cerebral Myelination

Myelin basic protein (MBP) is one of the most abundant proteins in cerebral white matter, and helps to maintain the correct structure of myelin. Neurofilament heavy chain (NfH) is a neurofilament that contributes to the growth and stability of axons. NfH and MBP are considered axon-specific biomarkers [12], which are generally used in combination to identify white matter axons and wrapped myelin. In this study, immunofluorescence staining was performed for MBP and NfH to facilitate the overview of myelination in periventricular white matter, since it is the most studied anatomical structure involved in preterm brain injury. The fixed brain tissues were embedded with OCT after dehydration with a 20 g/L sucrose solution, and then cut into 8-µm-thick sections. The frozen sections were washed with PBS, blocked with 5% donkey serum, and probed with primary antibodies as follows: mouse anti-mouse MBP antibody (808402, BioLegend, San Diego, CA, USA, 1:100) and rabbit anti-mouse NfH antibody (ab207176, Abcam, Cambridge, UK, 1:1000). After incubation at 4 °C overnight for 16 h, the sections were probed with secondary antibodies as follows: donkey anti-rabbit Cy2 (111-225-003, Jackson, 1:500) and donkey anti-mouse Cy3 (715-165-151, Jackson, 1:500), then incubated at room temperature for 1 h. Then, the sections were stained with 4′,6-diamidino-2-phenylindole (DAPI) for 15 min and mounted with AAT Bioquest, followed by observation under laser scanning confocal microscopy. Pictures were taken at 100 times magnification (10 × ocular and 10 × objective). The parameters were set as follows: DAPI: laser line: 405 nm, PMT detector, gain: 696 V; Cy2: laser line 488 nm, PMT detector, gain: 805 V; Cy3: laser line 552 nm, HyD detector, gain 15%; exposure time: 12 s.

2.4. Western Blot of MBP and GFAP

As described above, MBP is the most important biomarker of myelin. So, western blot analysis was performed to quantify MBP expression. Glial fibrillary acidic protein (GFAP) is a biomarker for astrocytes [13]. Astrocytes outnumber neurons in human neocortical white matter, and they are vulnerable and responsive to injury. Once encountered with injury, GFAP increases in astroglial cells and processes [14], which is considered a sensitive indicator of brain injury. So, western blot was also performed to quantify GFAP expression. Total protein was extracted using tissue protein extraction reagent (78510, Thermo, Waltham, MA, USA) mixed with a Protease Inhibitor Cocktail (87785, Thermo) under 99:1 proportion. Every 10 mg of brain tissue was added to 100 µL protein extraction reagent, and then ground in a tissue grinder at a rate of 60 Hz for 1 min. The ground mixture was placed on ice for 40 min, and then centrifuged at a refrigerated centrifuge at a rate of 14,000× *g* at 4 °C for 10 min. The supernatant was absorbed into a new Ep tube with a pipette and centrifuged again for 20 min. The final supernatant was transferred into the new Ep tube for analysis. The concentration of protein was confirmed using the bicinchoninic acid assay (BCA). In brief, the standard protein was diluted into 8 different concentrations by diluent to make the standard curve. The samples were diluted 50 times for measurement. The diluted standard protein and samples were added in 96-well plates with a total of 20 µL in each well (3 wells for each standard protein or sample). Exactly 200 µL of BCA working reagent was added to each well and incubated at 37 °C for 30 min. The 96-well plate was put into the Varioskan LUX Multimode Microplate Reader and measured at A562. The standard curve was drawn according to the concentrations of standard protein and their absorbance values. The concentrations of the samples were calculated according to the standard curve. Then, the protein samples were diluted to a uniform concentration by adding protein extraction reagent, and 5 × sodium dodecyl sulfate (SDS) loading buffer of 1/4 volume was added to adjust the final concentration to 5 μg/μL. The mixtures were denatured in a metal bath at 95 °C for 10 min. For western blot, a total of 20 μg of protein (4 μL) was loaded onto 12% SDS-polyacrylamide gels for electrophoresis and transferred onto polyvinylidene difluoride membranes. The membranes were blocked with 5% BSA in Tris-buffered saline-Tween (TBST) for 2 h, and incubated with primary rabbit anti-mouse antibodies: mouse anti-mouse MBP anti-body (808402, BioLegend, San Diego, CA, USA, 1:2000), rabbit anti-mouse GFAP (80788S, CST, Boston, MA, USA, 1:1000), GAPDH (bas 132004, Absin, Shanghai, China, 1:3000), and beta actin antibody (abs132001, Absin, 1:3000) at 4 °C overnight for 16 h. The membranes were then incubated with goat anti-rabbit IgG-HRP (abs20040, Absin, 1:5000) or goat anti-mouse IgG-HRP (abs20039, Absin, 1:5000) for 1 h. Protein blanks were visualized using super signal west femto maximum sensitivity (34096, Thermo) and photographed using a gel imaging system. Beta actin served as the internal reference, and the ratio of the gray value of the target protein to beta actin was used as the relative protein expression. The calculation of the gray value was performed using Image J software (Fiji, developed by NIH and LOCI, Bethesda, MD, USA).

2.5. Statistical Analysis

Statistical analysis was conducted using GraphPad Prism software. Descriptive data were presented as means ± SD. Survival rates were compared via a Log-rank test. Continuous variables were compared between two groups via 2-tailed Student's t test, including 6 samples in each group. A p value of <0.05 was considered as statistically significant.

3. Results

3.1. Persistent Alveolar Arrest during Neonatal Hyperoxia Exposure

A total of 6 litters of newborn mice were included in this study. At P0, there were 48 newborn mice without differences in body weight. Hyperoxia exposure decreased the survival rate of pups from P0 to P20 (Figure 1A).

At P10, HE staining showed that in the hyperoxia group, the size of alveoli enlarged, and the number of alveoli and secondary septa declined, while in the air group, secondary septa were abundant, which separated the alveolar sacs, resulting in smaller alveoli and an increased number of terminal alveoli (Figure 1B). Morphological assessment showed that RAC decreased, while MLI increased significantly in the hyperoxia group compared to the air group, which further reinforced the changes by quantifiable index (Figure 1C). At P15 and P20, the enlargement of alveoli became more obvious, with a persistent decline of alveoli and secondary septa. This lung morphology was similar to that of an earlier stage of lung development, and could thus be described as alveolar arrest. These results definitely supported that hyperoxia caused developmental disturbances on the immature lung.

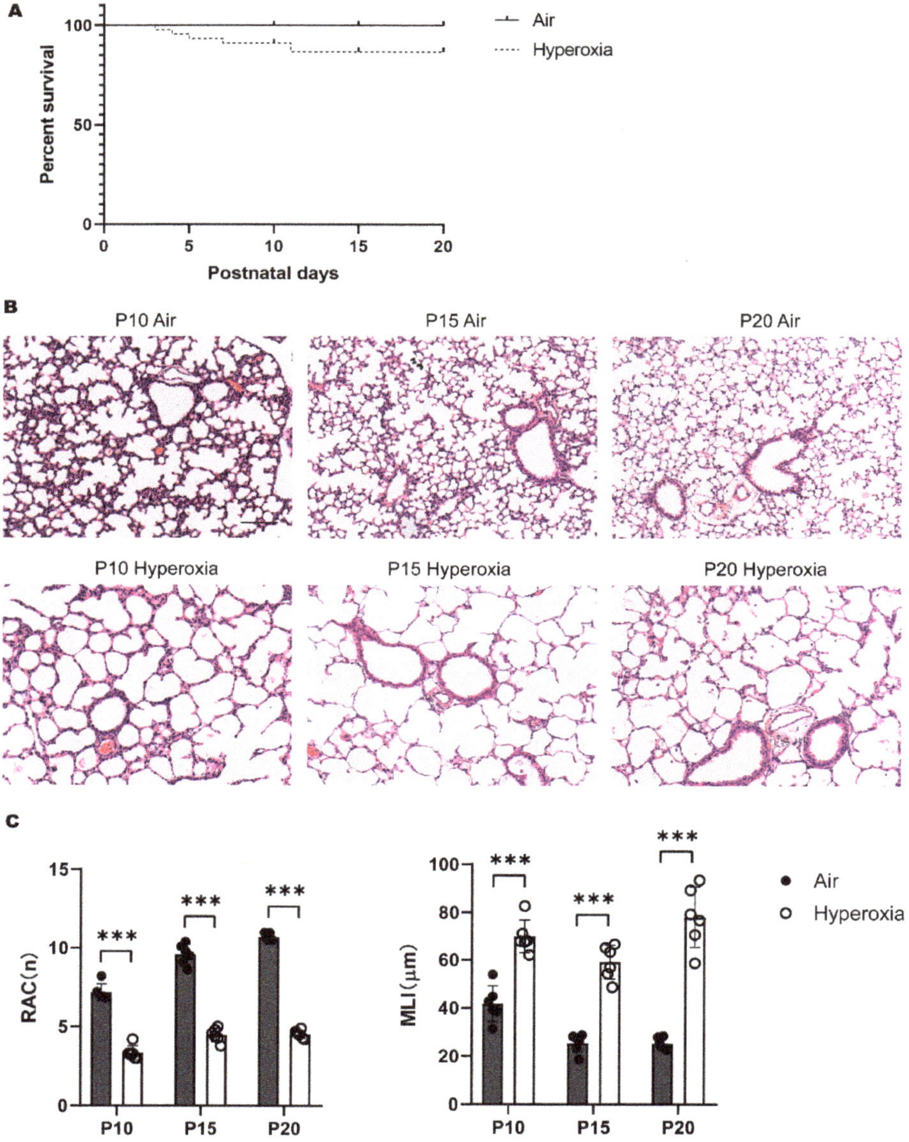

Figure 1. (**A**): Percentage survival of mice after 20 days of room air or 80% O_2 exposure ($p = 0.0184$). (**B**): Lung morphology at P10, P15, and P20, HE staining. The hyperoxia group showed less alveoli and enlarged alveolar space at P10, and sustained to P20. All the pictures were set on the same scale. Scale bar 100 μm. (**C**): Radial alveolar count (RAC) and mean linear intercept (MLI) counts and statistical graph. The hyperoxia group displayed decreased RAC and increased MLI. Data were calculated of six samples per group and presented as mean ± SD. *** $p < 0.001$.

3.2. Transient Myelination Impairment during Neonatal Hyperoxia Exposure

To access the myelination, we examined the expression of MBP (myelin basic protein, a major myelin protein) in the brain tissues through quantitative analysis by western bolt analysis combined with GFAP and qualitative display by immunofluorescence, combined with NfH. Western blot analysis showed that MBP was significantly lower in the hyperoxia group at P10 compared to the air group; at P15 MBP, it was raised to a comparable level as the air group, and at P20 MBP, it did not differ significantly in both hyperoxia and air groups (Figure 2A,B). The results indicated that cerebral myelination in the immature brain was impaired by hyperoxia. To reinforce hyperoxia-induced brain injury, we also examined the expression of GFAP (glial fibrillary acidic protein, a marker of astrocytes in the brain tissues). Western blot showed that GFAP increased significantly in the hyperoxia group at P10 compared to the air group, and the difference sustained to P15 and P20 (Figure 2A,B). The immunofluorescence showed corresponding dyeing of MBP and NfH in the corpus callosum (Figure 3). At P10, neurofibrillary dyed as green and red was thinner in the hyperoxia group than in the air group, and at P15 and P20, the neurofibrillary seemed to be the same thickness in both hyperoxia and air groups. These results provided direct molecular evidence of a negative effect of hyperoxia on the process of myelination. Myelination was frustrated with the decline of MBP and the elevation of GFAP at the early stage of the brain development. Although MBP was restored later, GFAP elevation continued. Cerebral myelination was impaired by hyperoxia at a critical developmental period, and left molecular evidence of persistent damage.

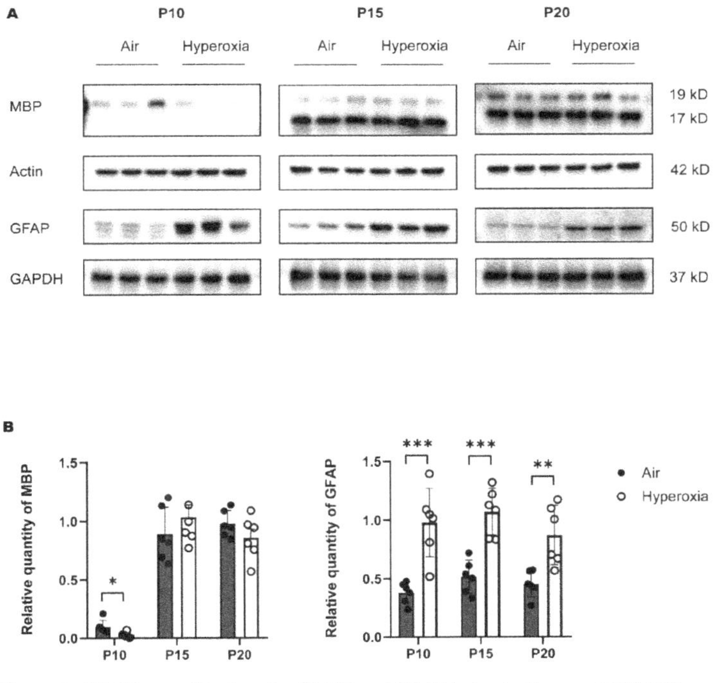

Figure 2. (**A**): Western blot bands of MBP and GFAP in brain tissues at P10, P15, and P20, showing the bands of MBP in the hyperoxia group were lighter than that in the air group at P10, while the bands of GFAP in the hyperoxia group were deeper than that in the air group at P10, P15, and P20. (**B**): Relative quantity of MBP equal to actin, and GFAP equal to GAPDH, showing the difference in MBP between the hyperoxia and air group at P10 was significant, while the differences in GFAP between the two groups at P10, P15, and P20 were significant. Data were calculated of six samples per group and presented as mean ± SD. * $p < 0.05$, ** $p < 0.01$, *** $p < 0.001$.

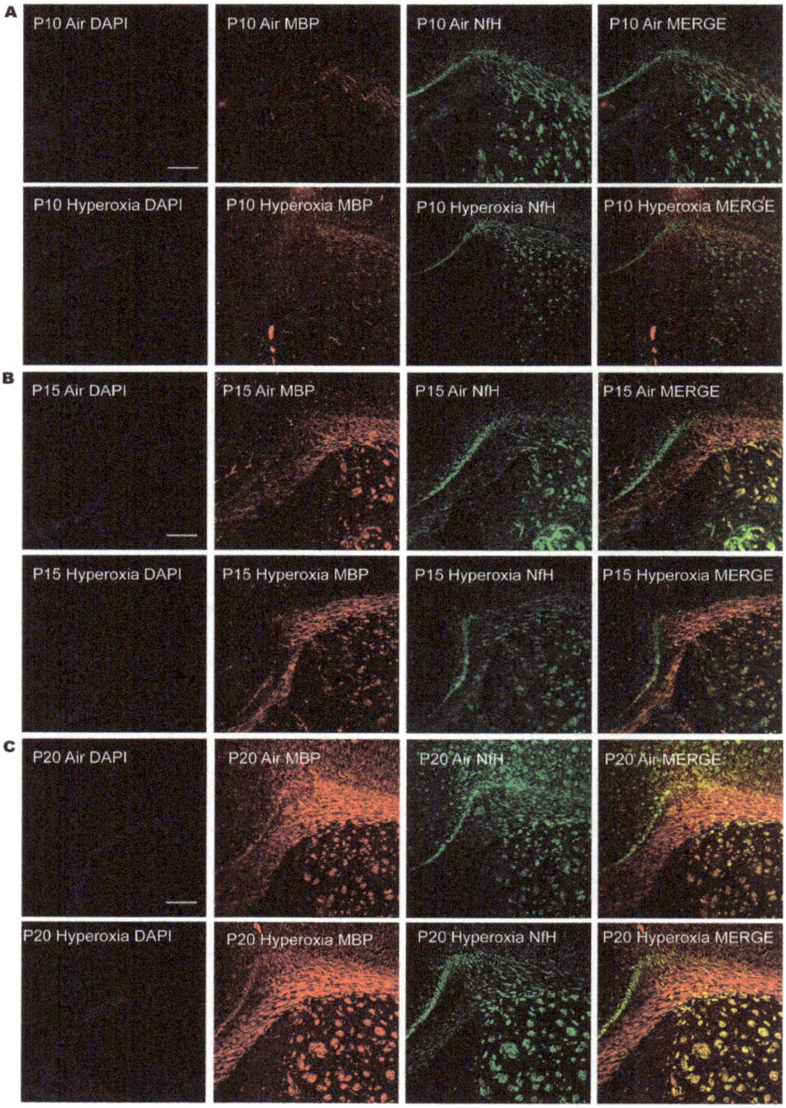

Figure 3. Immunofluorescence staining of MBP (red) and NfH (green) in periventricular white matter at P10 (**A**), P15 (**B**), and P20 (**C**), showing that MBP was inadequate at P10, but became abundant at P15 and P20. During postnatal hyperoxia exposure, MBP declined at P10 in the hyperoxia group, but was restored to the comparable as the air group. All the pictures were set on the same scale. Scale bar 50 μm.

4. Discussion

White matter lies beneath the gray matter cortex, which is composed of millions of bundles of axons (nerve fibers) that connect neurons in different brain regions into functional circuits [15]. The white color derives from the electrical insulation, which is called myelin, that enwraps axons. Myelination is the process of these myelin sheaths' formation. Myelin sheaths act to increase the conduction velocity of electrical impulses and improve brain connectivity [16]. Learning a new skill is associated with altered white matter structure, and the damage of white matter will cause impairments in sensory, motor, and cognitive functions [17]. In humans, myelination starts in mid-to-late gestation, which is equivalent to the perinatal and early postnatal ages in rodents [18]. In other words, the analogous time quantum of active myelination in rodents is around P2 to P10, which is congruent with the time preterm infants are born and survive, beginning from around 24–40 gestational age to 2–3 years after birth. In this time period, myelination is incomplete universally and develops dynamically. This critical time quantum was covered in our study, and the total expression of MBP can represent the overall degree of myelination in the brain. As shown definitely in our study, hyperoxia imposed a negative effect on myelination at P10 in rodents, equivalent to postnatal periods of preterm infants and their early childhood. Before this time period, neurons are established, but very few of the axons in the brain have been already myelinated, so communicational signals could barely transfer through neurons without myelin. The evolving myelination of white matter in this critical period contributes to pronounced improvements in cognitive abilities due to more rapid neural communication and integration of the signals across different brain regions involving well-recognized functions, such as vision [19], sensorimotor [20], memory [21], and language [22]. Infants receiving excessive and prolonged oxygen therapy during this period might experience deficits in myelination, resulting in the loss of approach through which signals contact [23]. The decline of MBP also indicated suppressed oligodendrogenesis, a process in which axon-myelinating oligodendrocytes recruit and generate MBP. In general, myelinating oligodendrocytes are differentiated from oligodendrocyte progenitor cells (OPCs), but they fail to differentiate in hyperoxia-induced brain injury due to degeneration and maturation arrest, thus ultimately resulting in frustrated myelination. As myelin matured, the difference in MBP expression between the hyperoxia and air group became inconspicuous at P15 and P20, which was a slow or quiet time since myelination is almost complete, equivalent to adulthood in humans. It was interesting that the observed micro quantificational changes of MBP did not sustain into adulthood. A speculated reason might be that an acceleration in the developmental trajectory of myelination would have happened in the healing process following hyperoxia injury. There is a potential backup pool of OPCs during adulthood, which are ready for myelin regeneration after injury [24,25]. Furthermore, OPCs are more resistant to oxidant stress in more mature bodies [26], so the decline of MBP caught up. However, MBP is not only the structural protein of myelin, but also an integral driver for myelin compaction via actin disassembly during myelin wrapping [27,28]. Although oligodendrocytes could survive and continue to express myelin genes in response to injury, they fail to maintain compacted myelin sheaths [29]. The compensation of MBP production through an excess of OPCs being generated after injury might not be integrated into neural circuits, thus causing failure in myelin remodeling [30]. Chang JL et al. demonstrated that hyperoxia caused abnormal myelin sheath formation and resulted in impaired myelin integrity, which contributed to WMI [31]. On the other hand, changes in the early developmental period may also play a role in the pathogenesis of EoP, with attention deficit and hyperactivity disorder, anxiety, and autism spectrum disorder as the most prevalent patterns, even absent of visible structural anomalies in the later life [32]. Khanbabaei M et al. also proposed that an altered developmental trajectory rather than structural anomaly could also be an important component of the etiology of EoP, especially those that referred to a milder degree of neurological impairment affecting mostly cognitive function and an increased risk of psychological disorders later in life [33]. It is not uncommon that children with social disorders have insignificant lesions in MRI imaging [34]. As revealed by Allin M et al., there might be a striking pattern of enhanced growth of the corpus callosum in adolescents born very preterm making up for early deficits, and this acceleration represented a delay of the normal maturation process that might be associated with a neuropsychological outcome [35]. Similarly, Morken TS et al. found that the alterations in white matter development caused by perinatal injury were reversible with age, indicating a maturation delay of the white matter [36]. Of note, the short-term prominent deficits of myelination might translate into long-lasting subtle white matter alterations associated with cognitive impairment or psychological disorders, which dominate the phenotypes of EoP in childhood among preterm children.

Astrocytes are predominant non-neuronal cells in the central nerve system (CNS), providing support for neuronal development; the interaction of astrocytes with neural cells synergistically promotes myelination [37]. Astrocytes have long been considered the major inhibitor on CNS repair under harmful stimulus. Previous studies demonstrated that astrocytes could exert potent proinflammatory functions as their primary mode of action after CNS injury [38]. Evidence has shown that neonatal myelination deficits are associated with neuroinflammation that could cause OPCs degeneration brought by astrocytes [39], and this might persist into adulthood [40]. Nowadays, it is recognized that astrocytes also play important roles in CNS repair and remyelination [41]. As a response to injury, the neurotransmitter adenosine 5′-triphosphate (ATP) is released from axons and activates receptors on astrocytes, causing them to release a cytokine that promotes oligodendrocyte development and thus increases myelination. That is, astrocytes can have a priming negative effect on myelination in early injury, as well as participating in repair and recovery after the insult. However, in chronic WMI, the differentiation of offsetting regenerative late ligodendroctye progenitors (preOLs) was hindered in the diffuse astrogliotic lesions, which was known as preOLs maturation arrest with a failure to generate myelin [34]. The reactive astrogliosis usually marked CNS structural lesions, with the elevation of GFAP, which was released after injury as the most important structural protein, labeling extensive branching of astrocytes in white matter [42]. As shown in our study, the decreased MBP expression did not sustain with age and prolonged hyperoxia exposure, but the increased GFAP expression continued, indicating a lasting reactive astrogliosis induced by hyperoxia. The latter might probably result in glial scar formation. In human beings, necrotic lesions (microscopic cysts) in WMI could evolve into glial scars over the course of several weeks, which is a persistent hallmark of brain injury [34].

A dilemma in the explanation of BPD-associated EoP is that BPD infants might encounter intermittent hypoxia frequently due to their immature respiratory control and poor lung function, which could also contribute to WMI. What cannot be ignored is that in spite of continuous oxygen therapy, premature infants experience multiple episodes of hypoxemia [43]. It is well documented that intermittent hypoxia elicits oxidative stress responses that occur during the re-oxygenation period [44]. Several studies demonstrated that recurrent hypoxia or hypoxia-hyperoxia encounters augmented oxidative stresses that generated a robust non-myelination preOLs accumulation relative to lesions in white matter compared to a single episode of hypoxia or hyperoxia [45,46]. In this experimental hyperoxia BPD model, mice could survive without respiratory dysfunction, excluding the effect that might be caused by hypoxia. Previous studies had already demonstrated that mice in this hyperoxia model maintained normal arterial oxygen levels [7]. Hence, the negative impact on the cerebral myelination was confirmed to come from direct hyperoxia injury. This result provided the rationale to avoid excess oxygen in clinical practice. However, extremely preterm infants could seldom survive without oxygen therapy due to immature lung and respiratory control at birth and within early days postnatal, raising challenges for neonatologists guarding against hyperoxia while avoiding hypoxia [47]. Lung-protective ventilation strategies have been proposed as the most important component in the management of preterm infants, such as optimizing gas exchange via volume-targeted ventilation during mechanical ventilation (MV) if necessary, avoiding MV if possible, optimizing non-invasive respiratory support, and setting a SpO_2 target of 90–95% in monitoring by pulse oximetry [48]. An important concept must be kept in mind—avoiding both prolonged periods of hypoxia ($SpO_2 < 80\%$) and fluctuations in SpO_2 [49].

In this study, we demonstrated concomitant brain injury at the molecular level in a BPD murine model. The strength of this study was that the hyperoxia model we applied involved both lung and brain injuries that mimic preterm birth conditions well. The results provided a rational explanation of BPD-associated EoP based on molecular mechanisms. Molecular changes were dynamically inspected, which provided a panoramic understanding of the impact of hyperoxia on the developmental brain.

There were still several limitations in this study. First, whether the lung-brain axis acted in the development of lung and brain injury in this hyperoxia model was not considered. Second, although pathological changes in this hyperoxia animal model were typical, the clinical relevance of the results has to be interpreted with caution because of the differences in conditions where alveolarization and brain development take place between rodents and humans. In addition, this chronic hyperoxia-induced lung injury model may not necessarily mimic BPD [50]. Further research is needed to validate the findings in large animal models of prematurity, which will enable the improvement of clinical translation.

5. Conclusions

Neonatal hyperoxia exposure caused an arrest of lung development, as well as an obstacle of myelination process in the white matter of the immature brain, with a decline of MBP in the generation period of myelin and persistent astrogliosis.

Author Contributions: W.C. designed and performed the study, and wrote the draft. R.W. provided methods for the study. C.C. supervised the study and reviewed the manuscript. All authors have read and agreed to the published version of the manuscript.

Funding: This work was supported by funds from Children's Hospital of Fudan University and the Fujian Provincial Health Commission (Youth Project Funding 2020QNA078).

Institutional Review Board Statement: The animal study was conducted in animal care facilities at Fudan University Affiliated Pudong Medical Center, Shanghai, China (approval code: XYXKHU2020-0005, approval date: 9 April 2020). The study project was reviewed and approved by the Children's Hospital of Fudan University (approval code: 00033, approval date: 14 November 2022).

Informed Consent Statement: Not applicable.

Data Availability Statement: Data presented in this article are available on request from the corresponding author.

Conflicts of Interest: The authors declare no conflict of interest.

References

1. Silva, L.V.; De Araújo, L.B.; Azevedo, V.M.G.D.O. Assessment of the neuropsychomotor development in the first year of life of premature infants with and without bronchopulmonary dysplasia. *Rev. Bras. De Ter. Intensiv.* **2018**, *30*, 174–180. [CrossRef] [PubMed]
2. Choi, E.K.; Shin, S.H.; Kim, E.-K.; Kim, H.-S. Developmental outcomes of preterm infants with bronchopulmonary dysplasia-associated pulmonary hypertension at 18–24 months of corrected age. *BMC Pediatr.* **2019**, *19*, 26. [CrossRef] [PubMed]
3. Klein, L.; Van Steenwinckel, J.; Fleiss, B.; Scheuer, T.; Bührer, C.; Faivre, V.; Lemoine, S.; Blugeon, C.; Schwendimann, L.; Csaba, Z.; et al. A unique cerebellar pattern of microglia activation in a mouse model of encephalopathy of prematurity. *Glia* **2022**, *70*, 1699–1719. [CrossRef] [PubMed]
4. Jantzie, L.L.; Winer, J.L.; Maxwell, J.R.; Chan, L.; Robinson, S. Modeling Encephalopathy of Prematurity Using Prenatal Hypoxia-ischemia with Intra-amniotic Lipopolysaccharide in Rats. *J. Vis. Exp.* **2015**, *105*, 53196.
5. Ten, V.S. Mitochondrial dysfunction in alveolar and white matter developmental failure in premature infants. *Pediatr. Res.* **2016**, *81*, 286–292. [CrossRef] [PubMed]
6. Jungner, S.; Kvist, S.V.; Romantsik, O.; Bruschettini, M.; Ekström, C.; Bendix, I.; Herz, J.; Felderhoff-Mueser, U.; Bibic, A.; Zandt, R.I.; et al. White Matter Brain Development after Exposure to Circulating Cell-Free Hemoglobin and Hyperoxia in a Rat Pup Model. *Dev. Neurosci.* **2020**, *41*, 1–13. [CrossRef]
7. Lithopoulos, M.A.; Toussay, X.; Zhong, S.; Xu, L.; Mustafa, S.B.; Ouellette, J.; Freitas-Andrade, M.; Comin, C.H.; Bassam, H.A.; Baker, A.N.; et al. Neonatal hyperoxia in mice triggers long-term cognitive deficits via impairments in cerebrovascular function and neurogenesis. *J. Clin. Investig.* **2022**, *132*, e146095. [CrossRef]
8. Semple, B.D.; Blomgren, K.; Gimlin, K.; Ferriero, D.M.; Noble-Haeusslein, L.J. Brain development in rodents and humans: Identifying benchmarks of maturation and vulnerability to injury across species. *Prog. Neurobiol.* **2013**, *106–107*, 1–16. [CrossRef]
9. Nardiello, C.; Mižíková, I.; Silva, D.M.; Ruiz-Camp, J.; Mayer, K.; Vadász, I.; Herold, S.; Seeger, W.; Morty, R.E. Standardisation of oxygen exposure in the development of mouse models for bronchopulmonary dysplasia. *Dis. Model. Mech.* **2017**, *10*, 185–196. [CrossRef]

10. Cooney, T.P.; Thurlbeck, W.M. The radial alveolar count method of Emery and Mithal: A reappraisal 1--postnatal lung growth. *Thorax* **1982**, *37*, 572–579. [CrossRef]
11. Knudsen, L.; Weibel, E.R.; Gundersen, H.J.G.; Weinstein, F.V.; Ochs, M. Assessment of air space size characteristics by intercept (chord) measurement: An accurate and efficient stereological approach. *J. Appl. Physiol.* **2010**, *108*, 412–421. [CrossRef]
12. Bohnert, S.; Wirth, C.; Schmitz, W.; Trella, S.; Monoranu, C.-M.; Ondruschka, B.; Bohnert, M. Myelin basic protein and neurofilament H in postmortem cerebrospinal fluid as surrogate markers of fatal traumatic brain injury. *Int. J. Leg. Med.* **2021**, *135*, 1525–1535. [CrossRef]
13. Brenner, M.; Messing, A. Regulation of GFAP Expression. *ASN Neuro* **2021**, *13*, 1759091420981206. [CrossRef] [PubMed]
14. Colombo, J.A.; Yáñez, A.; Lipina, S.J. Interlaminar astroglial processes in the cerebral cortex of non human primates: Response to injury. *J. Fur Hirnforsch.* **1997**, *38*, 503–512.
15. Lebel, C.; Deoni, S. The development of brain white matter microstructure. *Neuroimage* **2018**, *182*, 207–218. [CrossRef]
16. Fields, R.D. Change in the Brain's White Matter. *Science* **2010**, *330*, 768–769. [CrossRef] [PubMed]
17. Buyanova, I.S.; Arsalidou, M. Cerebral White Matter Myelination and Relations to Age, Gender, and Cognition: A Selective Review. *Front. Hum. Neurosci.* **2021**, *15*, 662031. [CrossRef] [PubMed]
18. Zhang, S.; Wang, Y.; Xu, J.; Kim, B.; Deng, W.; Guo, F. HIFα Regulates Developmental Myelination Independent of Autocrine Wnt Signaling. *J. Neurosci.* **2021**, *41*, 251–268. [CrossRef] [PubMed]
19. Rokem, A.; Takemura, H.; Bock, A.S.; Scherf, K.S.; Behrmann, M.; Wandell, B.A.; Fine, I.; Bridge, H.; Pestilli, F. The visual white matter: The application of diffusion MRI and fiber tractography to vision science. *J. Vis.* **2017**, *17*, 4. [CrossRef] [PubMed]
20. Ciccarelli, O.; Catani, M.; Johansen-Berg, H.; Clark, C.; Thompson, A. Diffusion-based tractography in neurological disorders: Concepts, applications, and future developments. *Lancet Neurol.* **2008**, *7*, 715–727. [CrossRef]
21. Benear, S.; Ngo, C.T.; Olson, I.R. Dissecting the Fornix in Basic Memory Processes and Neuropsychiatric Disease: A Review. *Brain Connect.* **2020**, *10*, 331–354. [CrossRef]
22. Friederici, A.D. White-matter pathways for speech and language processing. *Handb. Clin. Neurol.* **2015**, *129*, 177–186. [CrossRef]
23. Spaas, J.; van Veggel, L.; Schepers, M.; Tiane, A.; van Horssen, J.; Wilson, D.M.; Moya, P.R.; Piccart, E.; Hellings, N.; Eijnde, B.O.; et al. Oxidative stress and impaired oligodendrocyte precursor cell differentiation in neurological disorders. *Cell Mol Life Sci.* **2021**, *78*, 4615–4637. [CrossRef] [PubMed]
24. Kuhn, S.; Gritti, L.; Crooks, D.; Dombrowski, Y. Oligodendrocytes in Development, Myelin Generation and Beyond. *Cells* **2019**, *8*, 1424. [CrossRef]
25. Bacmeister, C.M.; Barr, H.J.; McClain, C.R.; Thornton, M.A.; Nettles, D.; Welle, C.G.; Hughes, E.G. Motor learning promotes remyelination via new and surviving oligodendrocytes. *Nat. Neurosci.* **2020**, *23*, 819–831. [CrossRef] [PubMed]
26. Hooft, J.V.; van der Lee, J.H.; Opmeer, B.C.; Aarnoudse-Moens, C.S.H.; Leenders, A.G.E.; Mol, B.W.J.; de Haan, T.R. Predicting developmental outcomes in premature infants by term equivalent MRI: Systematic review and meta-analysis. *Syst. Rev.* **2015**, *4*, 71. [CrossRef] [PubMed]
27. Zuchero, J.B.; Fu, M.-M.; Sloan, S.A.; Ibrahim, A.; Olson, A.; Zaremba, A.; Dugas, J.C.; Wienbar, S.; Caprariello, A.V.; Kantor, C.; et al. CNS Myelin Wrapping Is Driven by Actin Disassembly. *Dev. Cell* **2015**, *34*, 152–167. [CrossRef]
28. Brady, S.T.; Witt, A.S.; Kirkpatrick, L.L.; De Waegh, S.M.; Readhead, C.; Tu, P.-H.; Lee, V.M.-Y. Formation of Compact Myelin Is Required for Maturation of the Axonal Cytoskeleton. *J. Neurosci.* **1999**, *19*, 7278–7288. [CrossRef]
29. Meschkat, M.; Steyer, A.M.; Weil, M.-T.; Kusch, K.; Jahn, O.; Piepkorn, L.; Agüi-Gonzalez, P.; Phan, N.T.N.; Ruhwedel, T.; Sadowski, B.; et al. White matter integrity in mice requires continuous myelin synthesis at the inner tongue. *Nat. Commun.* **2022**, *13*, 1163. [CrossRef]
30. Ritter, J.; Schmitz, T.; Chew, L.-J.; Bührer, C.; Möbius, W.; Zonouzi, M.; Gallo, V. Neonatal Hyperoxia Exposure Disrupts Axon–Oligodendrocyte Integrity in the Subcortical White Matter. *J. Neurosci.* **2013**, *33*, 8990–9002. [CrossRef]
31. Chang, J.L.; Bashir, M.; Santiago, C.; Farrow, K.; Fung, C.; Brown, A.S.; Dettman, R.W.; Dizon, M.L. Intrauterine Growth Restriction and Hyperoxia as a Cause of White Matter Injury. *Dev. Neurosci.* **2018**, *40*, 344–357. [CrossRef]
32. Johnson, S.; Marlow, N. Preterm birth and childhood psychiatric disorders. *Pediatr. Res.* **2011**, *69 Pt 2*, 11–18. [CrossRef] [PubMed]
33. Khanbabaei, M.; Hughes, E.; Ellegood, J.; Qiu, L.R.; Yip, R.; Dobry, J.; Murari, K.; Lerch, J.P.; Rho, J.M.; Cheng, N. Precocious myelination in a mouse model of autism. *Transl. Psychiatry* **2019**, *9*, 251. [CrossRef] [PubMed]
34. Bs, J.R.B.; Maire, J.; Riddle, A.; Gong, X.; Nguyen, T.; Nelson, K.; Luo, N.L.; Ren, J.; Struve, J.; Sherman, L.S.; et al. Arrested preoligodendrocyte maturation contributes to myelination failure in premature infants. *Ann. Neurol.* **2012**, *71*, 93–109. [CrossRef]
35. Allin, M.; Nosarti, C.; Narberhaus, A.; Walshe, M.; Frearson, S.; Kalpakidou, A.; Wyatt, J.; Rifkin, L.; Murray, R. Growth of the Corpus Callosum in Adolescents Born Preterm. *Arch. Pediatr. Adolesc. Med.* **2007**, *161*, 1183–1189. [CrossRef] [PubMed]
36. Morken, T.S.; Nyman, A.K.G.; Sandvig, I.; Torp, S.H.; Skranes, J.; Goa, P.E.; Brubakk, A.-M.; Widerøe, M. Brain Development after Neonatal Intermittent Hyperoxia-Hypoxia in the Rat Studied by Longitudinal MRI and Immunohistochemistry. *PLoS ONE* **2013**, *8*, e84109. [CrossRef] [PubMed]
37. Kıray, H.; Lindsay, S.L.; Hosseinzadeh, S.; Barnett, S.C. The multifaceted role of astrocytes in regulating myelination. *Exp. Neurol.* **2016**, *283 Pt B*, 541–549. [CrossRef]
38. Li, M.; Li, Z.; Yao, Y.; Jin, W.-N.; Wood, K.; Liu, Q.; Shi, F.-D.; Hao, J. Astrocyte-derived interleukin-15 exacerbates ischemic brain injury via propagation of cellular immunity. *Proc. Natl. Acad. Sci. USA* **2017**, *114*, E396–E405. [CrossRef]

39. Hagberg, H.; Mallard, C.; Ferriero, D.M.; Vannucci, S.J.; Levison, S.W.; Vexler, Z.S.; Gressens, P. The role of inflammation in perinatal brain injury. *Nat. Rev. Neurol.* **2015**, *11*, 192–208. [CrossRef]
40. Graf, A.E.; Haines, K.M.; Pierson, C.R.; Bolon, B.N.; Houston, R.H.; Velten, M.; Heyob, K.M.; Rogers, L.K. Perinatal inflammation results in decreased oligodendrocyte numbers in adulthood. *Life Sci.* **2014**, *94*, 164–171. [CrossRef]
41. Barnett, S.C.; Linington, C. Myelination. *Neurosci.* **2013**, *19*, 442–450. [CrossRef] [PubMed]
42. Jurga, A.M.; Paleczna, M.; Kadluczka, J.; Kuter, K.Z. Beyond the GFAP-Astrocyte Protein Markers in the Brain. *Biomolecules* **2021**, *11*, 1361. [CrossRef] [PubMed]
43. Ratner, V.; Slinko, S.; Utkina-Sosunova, I.; Starkov, A.; Polin, R.A.; Ten, V.S. Hypoxic Stress Exacerbates Hyperoxia-Induced Lung Injury in a Neonatal Mouse Model of Bronchopulmonary Dysplasia. *Neonatology* **2009**, *95*, 299–305. [CrossRef] [PubMed]
44. Martin, A.; Faes, C.; Debevec, T.; Rytz, C.; Millet, G.; Pialoux, V. Preterm birth and oxidative stress: Effects of acute physical exercise and hypoxia physiological responses. *Redox Biol.* **2018**, *17*, 315–322. [CrossRef]
45. Segovia, K.N.; McClure, M.; Moravec, M.; Luo, N.L.; Wan, Y.; Gong, X.; Riddle, A.; Craig, A.; Struve, J.; Sherman, L.S.; et al. Arrested oligodendrocyte lineage maturation in chronic perinatal white matter injury. *Ann. Neurol.* **2008**, *63*, 520–530. [CrossRef]
46. Ratner, V.; Kishkurno, S.V.; Slinko, S.K.; Sosunov, S.A.; Sosunov, A.A.; Polin, R.A.; Ten, V.S. The Contribution of Intermittent Hypoxemia to Late Neurological Handicap in Mice with Hyperoxia-Induced Lung Injury. *Neonatology* **2007**, *92*, 50–58. [CrossRef]
47. Davidson, L.M.; Berkelhamer, S.K. Bronchopulmonary Dysplasia: Chronic Lung Disease of Infancy and Long-Term Pulmonary Outcomes. *J. Clin. Med.* **2017**, *6*, 4. [CrossRef]
48. Muehlbacher, T.; Bassler, D.; Bryant, M.B. Evidence for the Management of Bronchopulmonary Dysplasia in Very Preterm Infants. *Children* **2021**, *8*, 298. [CrossRef]
49. Tana, M.; Tirone, C.; Aurilia, C.; Lio, A.; Paladini, A.; Fattore, S.; Esposito, A.; De Tomaso, D.; Vento, G. Respiratory Management of the Preterm Infant: Supporting Evidence-Based Practice at the Bedside. *Children* **2023**, *10*, 535. [CrossRef]
50. Giusto, K.; Wanczyk, H.; Jensen, T.; Finck, C. Hyperoxia-induced bronchopulmonary dysplasia: Better models for better therapies. *Dis. Model. Mech.* **2021**, *14*, dmm047753. [CrossRef]

children

MDPI

Article

Disparities in Neonatal Mortalities in the United States

Ibrahim Qattea [1,2,*], Maria Burdjalov [3], Amani Quatei [1], Khalil Tamr Agha [4], Rayan Kteish [2] and Hany Aly [1]

1 Department of Neonatology, Cleveland Clinic Children's, 9500 Euclid Avenue #M31-37, Cleveland, OH 44195, USA; iqattea@gmail.com (A.Q.); alyh@ccf.org (H.A.)
2 Department of Pediatrics, Nassau University Medical Center, New York, NY 11554, USA; rayankteish@gmail.com
3 College of Arts and Sciences, The Ohio State University, Columbus, OH 43210, USA; burdjalov.3@buckeyemail.osu.edu
4 Department of Pediatrics, Upstate Golisano Children Hospital, Syracuse, NY 13210, USA; khalil1986@windowslive.com
* Correspondence: dribrahimqattea@gmail.com; Tel.: +1-2165075509

Abstract: Objective: We aimed to look for the mortality of Black and White Neonates and compare the Black and White neonates' mortalities after stratifying the population by many significant epidemiologic and hospital factors. Design/Method: We utilized the National Inpatient Sample (NIS) dataset over seven years from 2012 through 2018 for all neonates ≤ 28 days of age in all hospitals in the USA. Neonatal characteristics used in the analysis included ethnicity, sex, household income, and type of healthcare insurance. Hospital characteristics were urban teaching, urban non-teaching, and rural. Hospital location was classified according to the nine U.S. Census Division regions. Results: Neonatal mortality continues to be higher in Black populations: 21,975 (0.63%) than in White populations: 35,495 (0.28%). Government-supported health insurance was significantly more among Black populations when compared to White (68.8% vs. 35.3% $p < 0.001$). Household income differed significantly; almost half (49.8%) of the Black population has income ≤ 25th percentile vs. 22.1% in White. There was a significant variation in mortality in different U.S. locations. In the Black population, the highest mortality was in the West North Central division (0.72%), and the lower mortality was in the New England division (0.51%), whereas in the White population, the highest mortality was in the East South-Central division (0.36%), and the lowest mortality was in the New England division (0.21%). Trend analysis showed a significant decrease in mortality in Black and White populations over the years, but when stratifying the population by sex, type of insurance, household income, and type of hospital, the mortality was consistently higher in Black groups throughout the study years. Conclusions: Disparities in neonatal mortality continue to be higher in Black populations; there was a significant variation in mortality in different U.S. locations. In the Black population, the highest mortality was in the West North Central division, and the lower mortality was in the New England division, whereas in the White population, the highest mortality was in the East South Central division, and the lowest mortality was in the New England division. There has been a significant decrease in mortality in Black and White populations over the years, but when stratifying the population by many significant epidemiologic and hospital factors, the mortality was consistently higher in Black groups throughout the study years.

Keywords: NICU; neonatal mortalities; survival; racial disparities; perinatal epidemiology

1. Introduction

Racial and ethnic disparities in neonatal mortality are an ongoing healthcare concern [1–3]. Ethnic disparities are not specific to the United States; other countries demonstrate a similar pattern for increased mortality in minority groups. For example, neonatal mortality in the United Kingdom is significantly higher in infants born to non-U.K. mothers when compared to infants born to U.K.-born mothers [1,2].

The annual reports by the Centers for Disease Control and Prevention (CDC) demonstrated ethnic disparity in mortality of infants < 1 year of age. The findings of several studies were consistent with CDC reports [1,4,5]. These reports are informative in monitoring the extent and progress of ethnic disparities in infant mortality in the United States. However, multiple unmet needs require studying.

In practically all age groups, the United States exceeded the Healthy People 2020 goals for a 10% reduction in baby and adolescent mortality by 2015. Reductions in baby congenital abnormalities and SIDS are the main causes of decline. Additionally, long-standing racial/ethnic disparities in the United States still exist; in 2015, mortality rates were higher for Black populations than for White populations across all age groups, including for young adults, where White mortality rates did not change. Long-standing social and economic inequality, which affects patient access to care, the standard of care, and doctors' and patients' attitudes toward care, is the cause of these disparities [6].

To advise a plan that mitigates contributing factors to ethnic disparity, it would be beneficial to stratify infant mortality into neonatal mortality in the first 28 days of life and post-neonatal infant mortality for infants dying after 28 days of life. Identifying epidemiologic and clinical characteristics of hospitalized neonates associated with mortality is critical for decreasing disparities. Establishing a trend analysis for mortality can provide actual information on the progress of ethnic disparity. Although the variations in neonatal mortalities across ethnic groups are known [7], the relationship of neonatal mortality with household income, type of healthcare insurance, type of birthing hospital, and other demographic and clinical characteristics is unknown.

In this study, we aimed to compare the mortality of Black and White neonates after stratifying the population by significant epidemiologic and hospital factors. We utilized the National Inpatient Sample (NIS) dataset from 1 January 2012 through 31 December 2018. We hypothesized that ethnic disparity exists for neonatal mortality similar to that reported in infant mortality by CDC. Moreover, the ethnic disparity in neonatal mortality continues after controlling for significant epidemiologic and hospital factors.

2. Methods

2.1. Data Sources and Management

This study utilized the de-identified National Inpatient Sample (NIS) dataset from the Healthcare Cost and Utilization Project (HCUP) from the Agency for Healthcare Research and Quality (AHRQ) during the period 1 January 2012 through 31 December 2018. HCUP contains the largest collection of hospital discharge data in the United States. The NIS dataset includes 20% of the HCUP samples weighted to represent 100% of all inpatients in the U.S. Each year, more than seven million cases are drawn from thousands of hospitals across the United States with various care levels (primary–tertiary), types of insurance (public or private), sizes of hospital (small, medium, or large), and many other demographic and clinical characteristics. The data have a variable for neonatal status, whether alive or dead. Data elements in the NIS are constructed in a uniform format with quality checks in place. The de-identified data do not need Ethics Committee or Institutional Review Board approval as no information or identification about the patients is present, and therefore, the study was waived from IRB. The NIS data are available online by HCUP from 1988 to 2018, thereby allowing for the analysis of trends over time. The weighted data contains more than 35 million hospitalizations nationally [8,9].

2.2. Study Design and Population

All inpatients with ages $\leq$ 28 days were identified during the study period. Records of neonates that were transferred from one facility to another were counted only at the referral center and not at the sending hospital to avoid duplication of records. Mortality rates were calculated and compared at different neonatal characteristics, hospital settings, and U.S. regions. In addition to ethnicity, neonatal characteristics used in the analysis included sex, household income, and type of healthcare insurance. Hospital characteristics were urban teaching, urban non-teaching, and rural. Hospital location was classified according to the 9 U.S. Census Division regions: New England, Middle Atlantic, East North Central, East South Central, West North Central, South Atlantic, West South Central, Mountain, and Pacific.

Binary analyses were conducted using the chi-square test. Regression analyses were conducted to control for confounding variables. Cochran–Armitage trend test was used to assess trends during the study years. Significance was considered when the *p*-value was <0.05. All analyses were performed on weighted data to represent the entire U.S. admission.

3. Results

A total of 27,408,250 inpatient neonates were identified during the study period. Duplicate records were identified in 471,820 neonates due to transfer among healthcare facilities; these were excluded. Among the 26,936,430 included neonates, there were 3,511,960 Black and 12,662,000 White. Other ethnicities that were not included in the analysis were Hispanic (n = 4,853,303) and Asian (n = 5,909,168).

Black neonates had 21,975 (0.63%) mortalities, whereas White neonates had 35,495 (0.28%) deaths, as shown in Figure 1. Sex distribution among Black neonates was 50.8% male and 49.2% females, and in White neonates was 51.4% males and 48.6% females. Government-supported health insurance was significantly more among Black neonates when compared to White neonates (68.8% vs. 35.3% $p < 0.001$). Household income differed significantly; almost half (49.8%) of the Black population has income $\leq$ 25th percentile for ZIP code compared to 22.1% in the White population, $p < 0.001$. Although most deliveries occurred in the South region for both Black and White populations, it was disproportionately higher in Black than White (58% vs. 39.6%, $p < 0.001$), Figure 2.

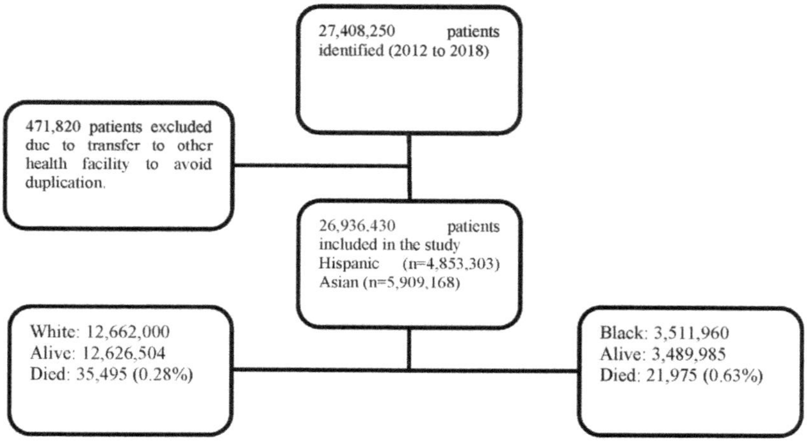

Figure 1. Study population algorithm.

Darker color represents higher mortality according to the range on each map.

- The upper map demonstrates neonatal mortalities in Black neonates.
- The lower map demonstrates neonatal mortalities in White neonates.

The solid line represents mortality in Black population. The dashed line represents mortality in White population. The upper panel represents postnatal mortality trends; mortality decreased significantly in Black and White neonates, ($Z = -3.26$, $p < 0.001$) and ($Z = -5.42$, $p < 0.001$), respectively. The lower panel represents neonatal mortalities according to sex. Black neonates had higher mortality than White in both sex groups ($p < 0.001$).

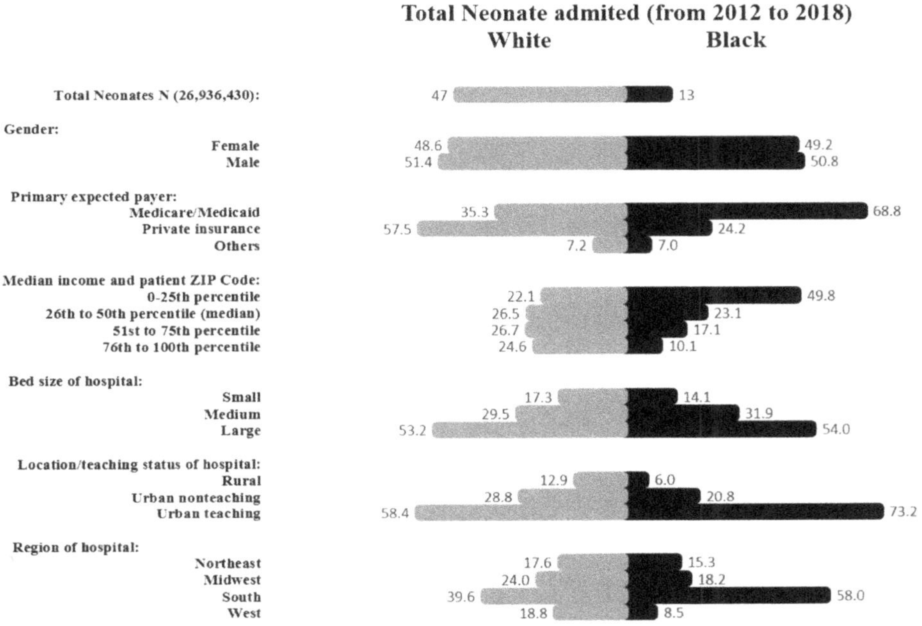

Figure 2. Characteristics of inpatient newborn admissions in Black and White populations. Data are expressed in percentages.

The upper panel represents neonatal mortality percentages trends in Black vs. White neonates according to the type of insurance. The solid line represents the mortality trend (%) for the Black neonates. The dashed line represents the mortality trend (%) for the White neonates. There was a significantly higher trend in Black mortalities when compared with Whites in all types of insurances, $p < 0.001$. The middle panel represents neonatal mortality percentages trends in Black vs. White neonates according to the household income according to the ZIP code. The solid line represents the mortality trend (%) for the Black neonates. The dashed line represents the mortality trend (%) for the White neonates. There was a significantly higher trend in Black mortalities when compared with Whites in all levels of income, $p < 0.001$. The lower panel represents neonatal mortality percentages trends in Black vs. White neonates according to the type of hospital. The solid line represents the mortality trend (%) for the Black neonates. The dashed line represents the mortality trend (%) for the White neonates. As previously mentioned, there was significantly higher mortality in the Black neonates when compared to Whites neonates in all types of hospitals, $p < 0.001$.

There was a significant variation in mortality in different U.S. locations. Maps for percentages of neonatal mortalities in different delivery locations are presented in Figure 3. These locations are categorized according to Census Division for Hospitals. In the overall population, the highest mortality was in the East South Central division (0.49%), and the lowest percentage of mortality was in the Pacific division (0.35%), $p < 0.001$. Black populations had the highest mortality in the West North Central division (0.72%), and their lowest mortality was in the New England division (0.51%), $p < 0.001$, whereas in the White populations, the highest mortality was in the East South Central division (0.36%), and the lowest mortality was in the New England division (0.21%) $p < 0.001$.

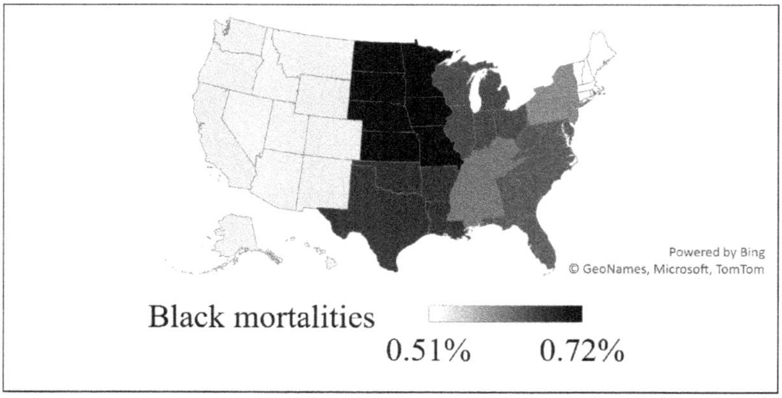

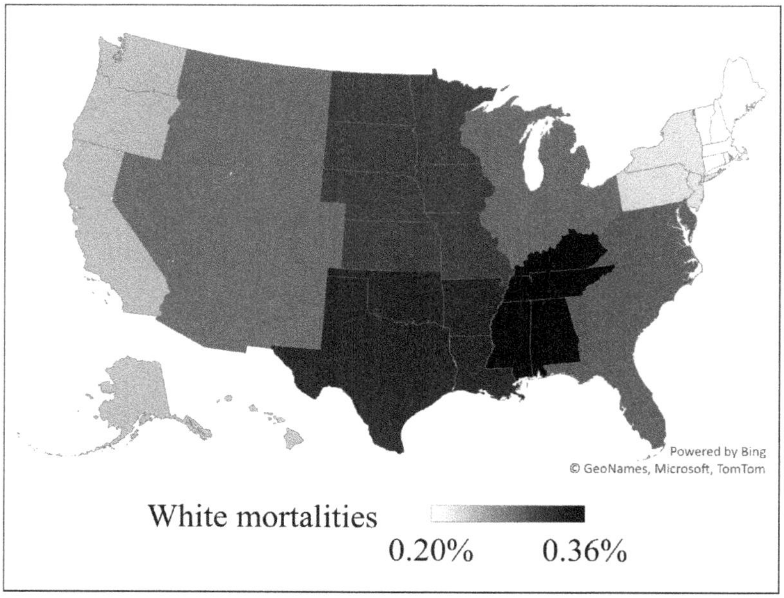

Figure 3. Delivery locations and neonatal mortalities percentages (regional percentages distribution of neonatal mortalities according to Census Division of Hospitals).

Trend analysis showed a significant decrease in mortality in Black and White populations over the years, ($Z = -3.26$, $p < 0.001$) and ($Z = -5.42$, $p < 0.001$), respectively. When stratifying the population by sex, mortality was consistently higher in Black populations in both sex groups throughout the study years (Figure 4).

After stratifying the population by type of insurance, mortality was higher in Black neonates compared to White neonates who had government-supported insurance (0.58% vs. 0.33%, $p \leq 0.001$), private insurance (0.57% vs. 0.22%, $p \leq 0.001$), and uninsured/self-paid (1.22% vs. 0.50%, $p \leq 0.001$). Trends for utilization of government-supported insurance in Black neonates and White neonates did not significantly change. Trends for uninsured/self-paid in Black and White neonates did not significantly change. Trends for mortality according to insurance type in government-supported population was not significant for decreased mortality in Black ($Z = -4.66$. $p < 0.2$) and in White neonates ($Z = -2.1$,

$p = 0.6$). For the privately insured population, there was no significant decrease in the Black ($Z = -2.6$. $p < 0.1$) and White neonates ($Z = -3.4$, $p = 0.13$). For uninsured/self-paid, there was a significant difference between the Black ($Z = -4.66$. $p < 0.0001$) and White neonates ($Z = -1.2$, p 0.03).

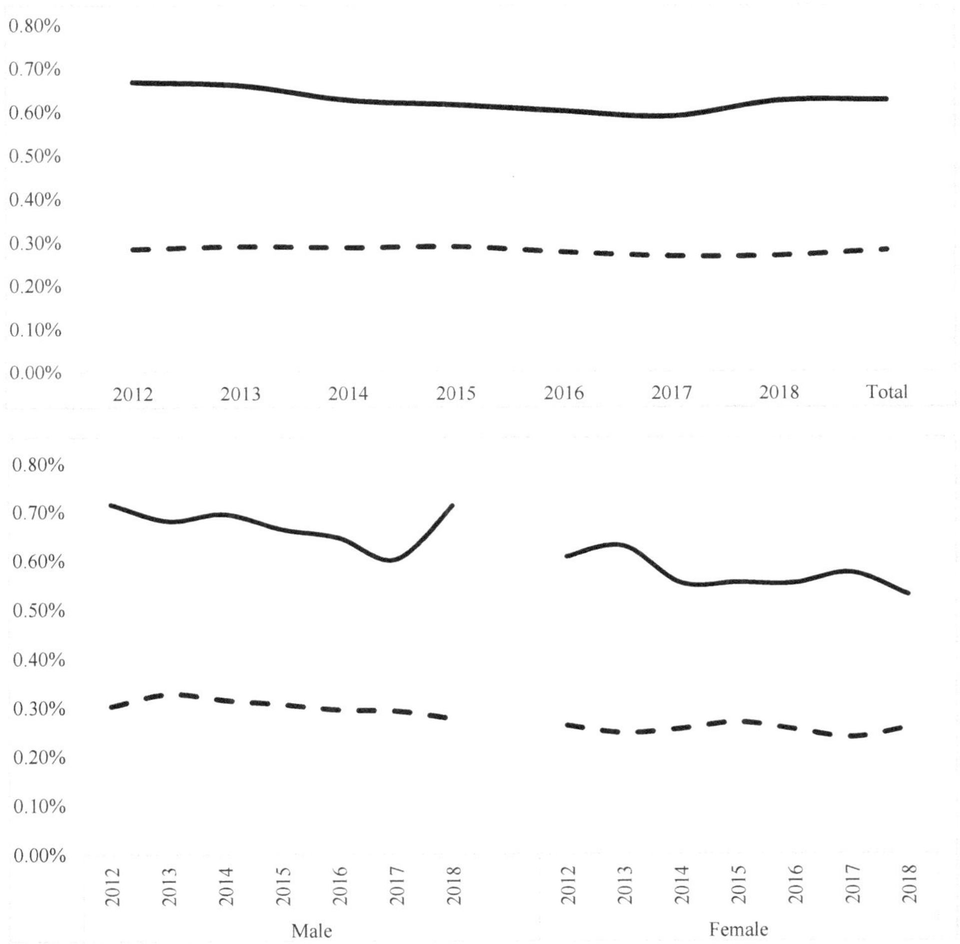

Figure 4. Trends for neonatal mortalities during the study period. The solid line represents mortality trend in Black neonates. The dashed line represents mortality trend in White neonates.

In trends for mortality among different household incomes according to zip code, there was a significantly higher number of Black mortalities when compared with Whites in all levels of income, $p < 0.001$ (Figure 5).

Trends in mortalities according to hospital type differed in Black vs. White. The solid line represents the mortality trend (%) for the Black neonates. The dashed line represents the mortality trend (%) for the White neonates. As previously mentioned, there was significantly higher mortality in the Black neonates when compared to Whites neonates in all types of hospitals, $p < 0.001$.

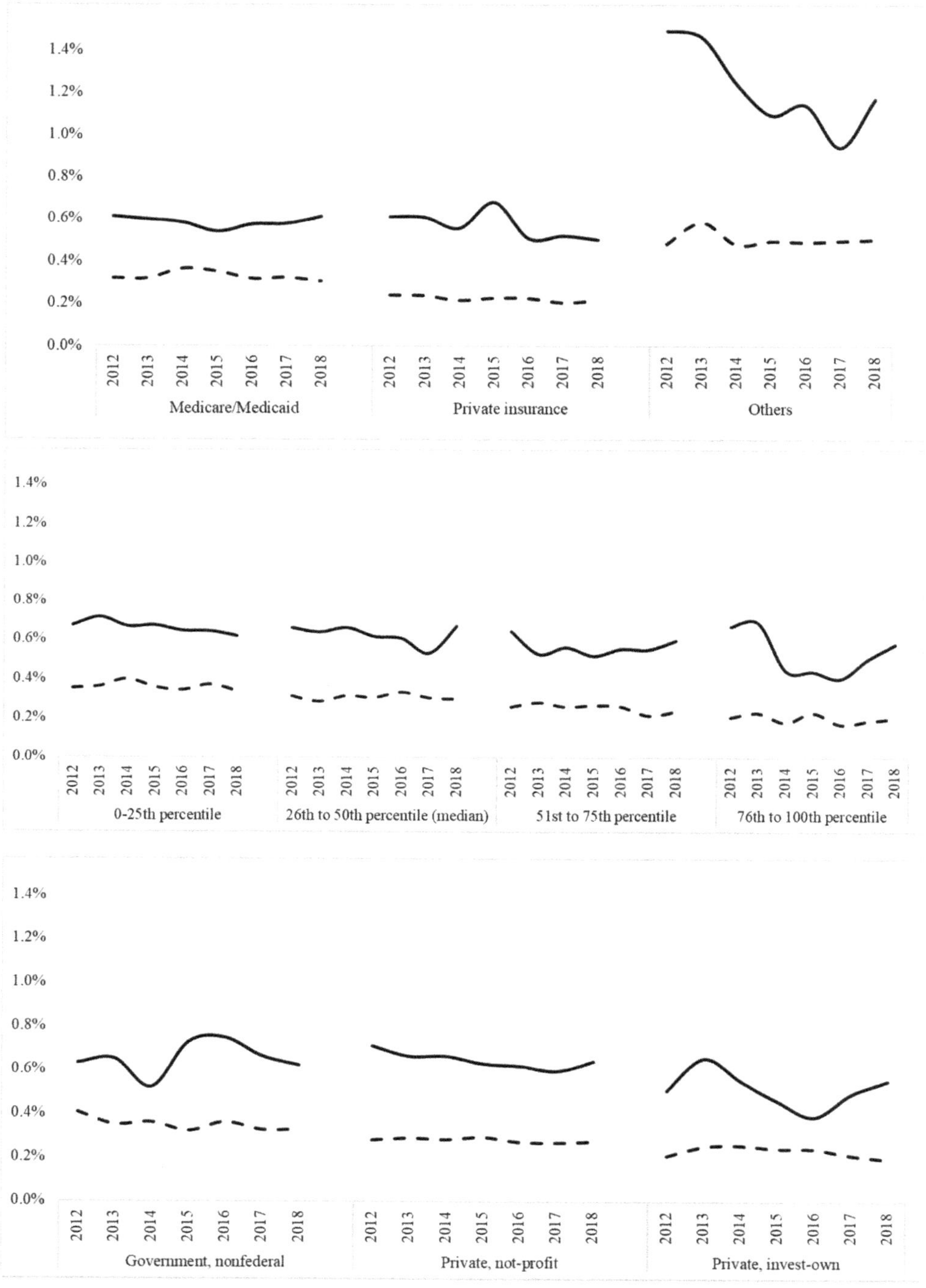

Figure 5. Trends for neonatal mortality percentages according to financial situations of patients and hospitals, Black vs. White neonates. The solid line represents mortality trend in Black neonates. The dashed line represents mortality trend in White neonates.

4. Discussion

Disparities in neonatal mortality continue to be higher in Black; number of mortalities in Black populations was 21,975 (0.63%) and in White was 35,495 (0.28%). Government-supported health insurance was significantly more among Black populations when compared to White (68.8% vs. 35.3% $p < 0.001$). Household income differed significantly; almost half (49.8%) of the Black population has income ≤ 25th percentile vs. 22.1% of White. There was a significant variation in mortality in different U.S. locations. In the Black population, the highest mortality was in the West North Central division (0.72%), and the lower mortality was in the New England division (0.51%), whereas in the White population, the highest mortality was in East South Central division (0.36%), and the lowest mortality was in the New England division (0.21%).

Trend analysis showed a significant decrease in mortality in Black and White populations over the years, but when stratifying the population by sex, type of insurance, household income, the type of hospital, the mortality was consistently higher in Black groups throughout the study years.

Trend analysis showed a significant decrease in mortality in the Black and White population over the years, and many studies demonstrated this finding even in the adult portion of the Black population [9,10]. The Black neonates always show the highest mortality in the U.S according to many studies; even some studies mentioned that the Black neonatal mortality rate is double the White mortality rate in the U.S. [11]. The novelty of our study is the stratification of the population by many significant epidemiologic and hospital factors. The Black neonates always show the highest mortality, and this study looks for many essential factors can contribute to the high Black mortality.

Disparities in maternal morbidity and mortality for Black women in the U.S. are the essential factor that impacts neonatal mortality and still exist in spit implementation of many systems for equity [12]. For example, racism may impact maternal health, mainly through discrimination among Black women as compared with White will significantly affect the perinatal care, and the neonatal outcome will be compromised at the end [13].

Neonatal mortality disparities may result from the many social, economic, and environmental exposures for pregnant Black women and neonates [14]. Other studies rely on many maternal factors, such as residential segregation, crime, inequality in income, suboptimal education, institutional racism, and built environment, which contribute to the poor outcomes of Black infants in the U.S. [3,15]. There are other factors as well, for example, abuses of Black American women by the medical system, inconsistent societal pressures on Black pregnant women, and historical stereotypes about Black women related to sexuality and pregnancy [16]. Finally, variations in neonatal mortality in the United States based on geographic location and the service available in the location of the Black community may contribute to variations in access to risk-appropriate delivery care [17].

Regardless, this study provides valuable insights into the disparities in neonatal mortality between Black and White populations in the United States. We still need to comprehend the underlying causes of these differences completely, and more research is necessary to create efficient solutions. More research is needed to understand how different hospital and epidemiological factors affect newborn mortality. Sex, insurance type, household income, and hospital type are a few examples of such factors. A fuller comprehension of how these characteristics interact with race and ethnicity will be essential to identify the most vulnerable populations. As well, researchers must examine the geographic variables causing these discrepancies, given the considerable range in mortality between U.S. locales. This may include variations in public health policy, socioeconomic situations, and healthcare access and quality by location. More longitudinal studies are required to monitor changes in newborn mortality over time and to evaluate the effectiveness of measures designed to lessen these inequalities.

Future research should concentrate on creating and evaluating policies and interventions to lower newborn mortality, particularly among Black communities. This could involve measures to lessen systematic racism in healthcare settings, alleviate socioeconomic inequalities, and increase access to high-quality healthcare.

This study has the strength of being the largest reported in the literature with a sample that exceeds 26 million infants that represent the entire United States, thereby eliminating the significant variation in practice and experience that is observed in currently available studies. In addition, the study could provide the national trend over the years for mortalities. The study inherited some limitations; this dataset is limited to the inpatient setting; therefore, long-term follow-up and mortality after hospital discharge are unavailable. We did not use ICD-9 and ICD-10, as the mortality is available in the dataset as a variable that makes the results more accurate.

Author Contributions: Conceptualization, I.Q., M.B. and H.A.; methodology, I.Q., M.B. and H.A.; software, I.Q. and M.B.; validation, I.Q., M.B. and H.A.; formal analysis, I.Q., M.B. and H.A.; investigation, I.Q., M.B. and H.A.; resources, I.Q. and M.B.; data curation, I.Q. and M.B.; writing—original draft preparation, I.Q., M.B., A.Q., R.K., K.T.A. and H.A.; writing—review and editing, I.Q., M.B., A.Q., R.K., K.T.A. and H.A.; visualization, I.Q., M.B., A.Q., R.K., K.T.A. and H.A.; supervision, H.A. All authors have read and agreed to the published version of the manuscript.

Funding: This research received no external funding.

Institutional Review Board Statement: Ethical review and approval were waived because the de-identified data do not need Ethics Committee or Institutional Review Board approval as no information or identification about the patients is present.

Informed Consent Statement: Patient consent was waived because the data is de-identified and no information or identification about the patients is present.

Data Availability Statement: The data available on the HCUP website: Purchase HCUP Data (ahrq.gov).

Conflicts of Interest: The authors declare no conflict of interest.

Abbreviations

Neonatal Mortalities; Survival; Racial Disparities; Perinatal epidemiology, NICU.

References

1. Chen, H.Y.; Chauhan, S.P.; Rankins, N.C.; Ananth, C.V.; Siddiqui, D.S.; Vintzileos, A.M. Racial and ethnic disparities in infant mortality in the United States: The role of gestational age. *Am. J. Perinatol.* **2013**, *30*, 469–475. [CrossRef]
2. Opondo, C.; Jayaweera, H.; Hollowell, J.; Li, Y.; Kurinczuk, J.J.; Quigley, M.A. Variations in neonatal mortality, infant mortality, preterm birth and birth weight in England and Wales according to ethnicity and maternal country or region of birth: An analysis of linked national data from 2006 to 2012. *J. Epidemiol. Community Health* **2020**, *74*, 336–345. [CrossRef] [PubMed]
3. Matoba, N.; Collins, J.W. Racial disparity in infant mortality. *Semin. Perinatol.* **2017**, *41*, 354–359. [CrossRef]
4. Infant Mortality | Maternal and Infant Health | Reproductive Health | CDC. 2021. Available online: https://www.cdc.gov/reproductivehealth/maternalinfanthealth/infantmortality.htm (accessed on 28 January 2022).
5. Alexander, G.R.; Kogan, M.; Bader, D.; Carlo, W.; Allen, M.; Mor, J.U.S. birth weight/gestational age-specific neonatal mortality: 1995-1997 rates for whites, hispanics, and blacks. *Pediatrics* **2003**, *111*, e61–e66. [CrossRef] [PubMed]
6. Khan, S.Q.; Berrington de Gonzalez, A.; Best, A.F.; Chen, Y.; Haozous, E.A.; Rodriquez, E.J.; Spillane, S.; Thomas, D.A.; Withrow, D.; Freedman, N.D.; et al. Infant and Youth Mortality Trends by Race/Ethnicity and Cause of Death in the United States. *JAMA Pediatr.* **2018**, *172*, e183317. [CrossRef] [PubMed]
7. Opondo, C.; Gray, R.; Hollowell, J.; Li, Y.; Kurinczuk, J.J.; Quigley, M.A. Joint contribution of socioeconomic circumstances and ethnic group to variations in preterm birth, neonatal mortality and infant mortality in England and Wales: A population-based retrospective cohort study using routine data from 2006 to 2012. *BMJ Open* **2019**, *9*, e028227. [CrossRef] [PubMed]
8. HCUP Sample Design: National Databases—Accessible Version. Available online: https://www.hcup-us.ahrq.gov/tech_assist/sampledesign/508_compliance/index508_2018.jsp#nisprior (accessed on 29 November 2021).
9. HCUP-US NIS Overview. Available online: https://www.hcup-us.ahrq.gov/nisoverview.jsp (accessed on 15 April 2022).
10. Buchanich, J.M.; Doerfler, S.M.; Lann, M.F.; Marsh, G.M.; Burke, D.S. Improvement in racial disparities in years of life lost in the USA since 1990. *PLoS ONE* **2018**, *13*, e0194308. [CrossRef] [PubMed]
11. Sosnaud, B. Cross-State Differences in the Processes Generating Black-White Disparities in Neonatal Mortality. *Demography* **2021**, *58*, 2089–2115. [CrossRef] [PubMed]

12. Noursi, S.; Saluja, B.; Richey, L. Using the Ecological Systems Theory to Understand Black/White Disparities in Maternal Morbidity and Mortality in the United States. *J. Racial Ethn. Health Disparities.* **2021**, *8*, 661–669. [CrossRef] [PubMed]
13. Minehart, R.D.; Bryant, A.S.; Jackson, J.; Daly, J.L. Racial/Ethnic Inequities in Pregnancy-Related Morbidity and Mortality. *Obstet. Gynecol. Clin. N. Am.* **2021**, *48*, 31–51. [CrossRef] [PubMed]
14. Willis, E.; McManus, P.; Magallanes, N.; Johnson, S.; Majnik, A. Conquering racial disparities in perinatal outcomes. *Clin. Perinatol.* **2014**, *41*, 847–875. [CrossRef] [PubMed]
15. Burris, H.H.; Hacker, M.R. Birth outcome racial disparities: A result of intersecting social and environmental factors. *Semin. Perinatol.* **2017**, *41*, 360–366. [CrossRef] [PubMed]
16. Rosenthal, L.; Lobel, M. Explaining racial disparities in adverse birth outcomes: Unique sources of stress for Black American women. *Soc. Sci. Med.* **2011**, *72*, 977–983. [CrossRef] [PubMed]
17. Lorch, S.A.; Rogowski, J.; Profit, J.; Phibbs, C.S. Access to risk-appropriate hospital care and disparities in neonatal outcomes in racial/ethnic groups and rural-urban populations. *Semin. Perinatol.* **2021**, *45*, 151409. [CrossRef] [PubMed]

children

MDPI

Article

What Mothers Know about Newborn Bloodspot Screening and the Sources They Use to Acquire This Knowledge: A Pilot Study in Flanders

Caroline di Gangi [1,†], Maren Hermans [1,†], Maissa Rayyan [2,3], François Eyskens [4] and Karel Allegaert [2,5,6,7,*]

1 Department of Public Health and Primary Care, Academic Centre for Nursing and Midwifery, 3000 Leuven, Belgium; digangicaroline@gmail.com (C.d.G.); maren.hermans@live.be (M.H.)
2 Department of Development and Regeneration, KU Leuven, 3000 Leuven, Belgium; maissa.rayyan@uzleuven.be
3 Neonatal Intensive Care Unit, University Hospitals, UZ Leuven, 3000 Leuven, Belgium
4 Centre for Metabolic Diseases, University Hospital Antwerp, University of Antwerp, 2650 Edegem, Belgium; francois.eyskens@uza.be
5 Department of Pharmaceutical and Pharmacological Sciences, KU Leuven, 3000 Leuven, Belgium
6 Leuven Child & Youth Institute, KU Leuven, 3000 Leuven, Belgium
7 Department of Hospital Pharmacy, Erasmus University Medical Center, 3015 GD Rotterdam, The Netherlands
* Correspondence: karel.allegaert@uzleuven.be; Tel.: +32-016-342020
† These authors contributed equally to this work.

Abstract: To learn what mothers know about newborn bloodspot screening (NBS), the procedure, and the sources used, a pilot study was performed. An online questionnaire was developed, with the first part focused on characteristics and the NBS procedure, and the second on knowledge, information sources, and health care providers (HCPs). This questionnaire was accessible until 200 answers were received. The characteristics of respondents were representative for the population. Mothers gave verbal consent in 69.5% of cases, 12.5% did not, and 18% stated that no consent was requested. The 'knowledge' part contained 12 closed questions, five multiple-choice questions on sources, and assessments (5-point Likert scores) of the information transfer. The mean knowledge level was 7.2/12. Screening concepts (consequences, likelihood, sensitivity, carrier) and absence of notification of normal findings were well known. The fact that NBS is not compulsory was poorly known, and post-analysis sample handling procedures were poorly understood. Key HCPs were midwifes (80.5%) and nurses (38.5%). When the leaflet (44%) was provided, the majority read it. Mean Likert scores were 3.36, 3.38, 3.11 and 3.35 for clarity, timing appropriateness, sufficiency, and usefulness. The knowledge level and consent practices were reasonably good. Key HCP were midwives and nurses, the leaflets were supporting. This should enable a quality improvement program to a sustainable NBS program in Flanders.

Keywords: newborn blood screening; knowledge; consent; mother; parent

1. Introduction

Newborn bloodspot screening (NBS) is one of the most-implemented population screening programs worldwide. While initially limited in terms of the number of diseases (phenylketonuria, hypothyroidism), NBS screening programs subsequently broadened their panel of conditions screened [1]. This was largely driven by technical improvements in diagnostics, and improved knowledge on disease mechanisms and history, converging with therapeutic interventions to improve the outcome in diagnosed infants. This progress relates to the fact that screening programs are driven by the criteria of Wilson and Jungner (an important health problem, the natural history of the condition is well understood, it is detectable at an early stage, earlier treatment should be beneficial, a suitable test should be available in this early stage (sensitivity/specificity), and the test should be acceptable) [1].

Although not causally related, this expansion of NBS programs also raised awareness of the shortcomings in parental education, information products, and the informed consent process. This can, in part, also relate to the fact that expansion of the NBS programs will also result in communications to the different stakeholders involved, and may induce reflections or questions. The provision of information to parents has been recognized as a crucial part of sustainable NBS programs, being that there is still lack of regulatory harmonization within Europe [2].

Almost all European countries provide information for parents (brochures, websites). About two-thirds of the countries ask for consent, while consent for long-term storage of blood spot cards is requested in a minority (30%) of European countries [1]. In a recent paper, Ijzebink et al. focused on these information products provided throughout Europe [3]. In this paper, 26 printed European products (like leaflets or flyers) were assessed on their content and knowledge, and rated according to a list of eight knowledge domains (screening purpose, false positive/negative findings, uncertainties and risks, medical implications, social implications, financial implications, follow-up, and support services). Despite some differences between European countries, most of these eight knowledge aspects were included in all information products, with most diversity related to the handling of residual bloodspot samples [3].

Along the same lines, the script for health care providers (HCPs) involved in NBS in Flanders (in the north of Belgium; the Dutch-speaking part) mentions the need to discuss the relevance of timely diagnosis, the importance of the postnatal age window (72–96 h) for screening, the practicalities related to the appointment for the screening (because of the short hospital stay after delivery), the need of verbal (concise) consent, and to make it clear that all initial screening costs are covered by the government, costs for additional tests after screening are reimbursed by the insurance, which diseases are screened for and, finally, the fact that NBS is not compulsory, but highly recommended [4]. In Flanders, long-term storage of the blood spot charts is not part of the program, and storage is limited to one year. These topics are also discussed in leaflets (printed, and as a downloadable pdf) and on a specific website (aangeboren.bevolkingsonderzoek.be) to inform both parents and the general public [5].

Informed consent necessitates that the relevant person(s) have been informed on the procedure and its potential consequences in such a way that it is reasonable to assume that the information has been understood sufficiently well to support their decision (irrespective of the subsequent decision itself) [6]. In the study by Frankova et al., 12/27 countries mentioned that checks (commonly based on surveys) are performed to verify that information indeed reaches the targeted populations [2]. In an attempt to obtain a first snapshot on what mothers know on NBS, and the sources they use in Flanders to acquire this knowledge (as the Flanders region or Belgium as a country were not included in European survey) [2], a pilot study was performed.

2. Materials and Methods

2.1. Perinatal Health Care Structures in Flanders and the Study Setting

Prenatal follow up in Flanders is mainly coordinated by obstetricians and midwives, with more limited involvement of general practitioners, and is still almost exclusively 'hospital'-driven. In 2021, there were 63,334 (64,282 births) deliveries in Flanders. Those deliveries almost exclusively occurred in one of the 59 hospitals ('maternities'), with about 0.8% of deliveries elsewhere (like at home, or in birth centers not connected to a hospital). In an attempt to evolve to a transmural care program, initiatives were taken to shorten the duration of hospitalization to 2–4 days, in part depending on the type of delivery. This shift has been facilitated by the development of midwife-driven home care programs, supported by general practitioners, obstetricians, and pediatricians [7,8]. Consequently, a relevant portion of newborns have their NBS screening performed at home by midwives, and different HCPs are commonly involved in the pregnancy and postpartum care.

Within this health care framework, and as a pilot study, we aimed to recruit 200 mothers who recently (maximum 1 year before the dissemination of the questionnaire) delivered in Flanders, understood Dutch sufficiently well to complete the questionnaire, were older than 18 years, and provided consent to contribute to the pilot study. We are aware that with this approach, partners of the mothers were a priori excluded. We are aware that this is a deficiency, but we deliberately had to do this to avoid 'dual' reporting within the framework and limitations of this pilot study.

2.2. Questionnaire

In the first part of the questionnaire, information on characteristics and background of respondents (like age, residency, primi- or multipara, level of education, place of delivery) and on the NBS procedure (collected yes/no), location (hospital or at home) of the procedure, consent recall) were collected. The second part focused on the knowledge itself, the sources of information used, and the HCPs involved. This part of the questionnaire was constructed in line with the approach described by Detmar et al. for a Dutch cohort, with some adaptations to the Flemish setting (health care organization, legal and regulatory environment, sources of information) [6]. To respect the methodology on questionnaire design, adaptations were initially made independently by CdG and MH, with subsequent cross-verification to attain consensus. In the event of absence of consensus, KA was involved. The final version was subsequently verified on face validity by these three authors.

2.3. Data Collection and Analysis

Questionnaires were distributed online (Qualtrics, Seattle, WA, USA), using social media platforms (Facebook, personal and group pages) and e-mail correspondence to nurseries. To assess the representativity of respondents, information on characteristics and background was compared to reference information on pregnancies in Flanders [7,9]. Data on the NBS procedure (collected yes/no, location of the procedure, consent recall) were more difficult to compare, as we could only retrieve a press release from the relevant agency that stated that 99% of the newborns undergo NBS in Flanders [10]. Data analysis on knowledge was based on maternal knowledge on the NBS procedure as the dependent variable; the independent variables were the information received (as perceived by the mother), parity (prima- versus multigravida), and the level of maternal education. We hereby a priori hypothesized that maternal knowledge would correlate positively with parity and the level of education.

2.4. Ethics, Privacy, and Data Management

The Ethics Committee Research of KU Leuven and University Hospitals Leuven approved the study protocol (MP022668, 5 December 2022, favorable advice). The questionnaire was preceded by an information letter, describing the aims of the study and the consent to contribute to the questionnaire. Consent to contribute and store responses for analysis (anonymous, confidential) was requested before the questionnaire could be completed.

3. Results

The final version of the 'knowledge' part (translated version, English, Table 1) contained 12 closed questions, and five multiple choice + open questions on the sources of information. We have provided the Dutch version of the questionnaire in a Supplemental Table S1 to facilitate future use.

Finally, based on a 5-point Likert score, respondents were requested to provide their assessment of the information transfer (clarity, appropriateness of timing, sufficiency, usefulness) process.

This questionnaire (characteristics and background, NBS procedure and knowledge part, and the general assessment of knowledge transfer process) was accessible online from 2 February 2023 to 18 April 2023, when 200 questionnaires were received.

Table 1. The final questionnaire.

Knowledge questions, closed
Diseases screened for with the NBS have severe consequences if not treated appropriately.
The likelihood that an infant has a disease screened for is low.
For the NBS, some blood is collected from the heel of the infant.
In the event of an abnormal NBS, additional investigations in the hospital are needed.
A normal NBS provides certainty that the infant is perfectly healthy.
The NBS test is reliable, as an infant with a given disease screened for will very likely be detected.
In the event of uncertainties, a second NBS is indicated.
The NBS is compulsory for any newborn.
A healthy person can still be the carrier of a genetic disease.
When the NBS is NORMAL, parents will NOT receive a notification.
Immediately after the NBS analysis, the blood sample will be destroyed.
Are you aware of the recent extension of diseases screened for with the NBS?
Knowledge questions, multiple choice, including open answers
Who was involved to inform you about the NBS (you can provide multiple answers)? (*midwife, nurse, obstetrician, general practitioner, information session during pregnancy, friends or peers, website 'aangeboren.bevolkingsonderzoek.be', television or radio, journals or magazines, the NBS folder, social media, I have not received information, others*)
What was the most relevant source of information on NBS for you (you can provide multiple answers)? (*midwife, nurse, obstetrician, general practitioner, information session during pregnancy, friends or peers, website 'aangeboren.bevolkingsonderzoek.be', television or radio, journals or magazines, the NBS folder, social media, I have not received information, others*)
If you have received the NBS folder, have you read this document? (*yes, I have read this document fully, partial, screened; no, as I was already aware of the folder, or I already knew on the NBS, not applicable as no folder received*).
Have you searched for other sources of information? (*no; yes, on the website 'aangeboren.bevolkingsonderzoek.be'; yes, on the internet, but other websites; yes, other folders, books or magazines; yes, I have discussed this with others; yes, as...*)
How do you overall assess the information you have received? (Likert score 0–5, where 0 is the worse score) (*clarity, appropriateness of the timing, sufficiency, usefulness*)

NBS: newborn bloodspot screening.

Participants were recruited by their own Facebook profiles (CdG, MH, n = 42), specific groups within Facebook (six groups, 709 messages, 100 participants), or nurseries (n = 79 nurseries contacted). Ninety-eight % of the participants finalized the questionnaire. To assess representativity of respondents to the Flemish pregnant and postpartum population, age, residence (postal code, provinces), parity, level of education, place of delivery (hospital, or out of hospital), collection of the NBS (yes/no; location (hospital/home)) of respondents were compared to the latest Perinatal Epidemiology Study Center (SPE) 2021 annual report and STATBEL report (education) (Table 2). Maternal age and place of delivery were similar, while there were some differences in place of residence, some overrepresentation in primigravidae, and respondents had a somewhat higher level of education compared to the reference population. Data on the NBS procedure (yes/no, place, verbal consent) were somewhat more difficult to compare with the reference population data, but also seem similar (Table 2). NBS were collected both in the hospital, as well as at home. Mothers recalled verbal consent in 69.5% of cases, 12.5% did not recall any consent request, and 18% stated that no consent has been requested.

Table 2. Representativity of the respondents to the Flemish pregnant and postpartum population (NBS: newborn blood screening) [8,9].

Variables	Categories	Respondents	Reference Population
Maternal age	<20 years	0.5%	0.9%
	20–24	13.5%	8.1%
	25–29	39%	32%
	30–34	34%	40.1%
	35–39	9%	15.4%
	≥40	4%	3.5%
Residence	Brussels	0.5%	unknown
	Brabant, Flemish	15%	14.4%
	Antwerp	28.5%	34.2%
	Limburg	34%	10.9%
	West Flanders	9%	17.4%
	East Flanders	13%	23.1%
Parity	Primipara	59%	45.2%
	Multipara	41%	54.8%
Education	Bachelor onwards	61.5%	56.2%
	≤High school	38.5%	43.8%
Place of delivery	Hospital	97%	96%
	Out of hospital	3%	4%
NBS collected	Yes	99%	>99%
	No	0.5%	
	Unclear	0.5%	
Place of NBS	Hospital	54%	unknown
	Home	46%	unknown

Based on the 12 questions provided, the mean level of knowledge was 7.2 (SD 2.4)/12, and 79% of the respondents had a score ≥6. The level of knowledge was correlated positively with the level of education, and without a difference between primi- and multipara. An overview on the responses to the individual questions is provided in Table 3.

The concepts of targeted screening (severe consequences, low a priori likelihood, sensitivity, carrier concept) and absence of notification in the event of normal findings are well known. In contrast, the fact that NBS is not compulsory in Flanders is only poorly known, and the post-analysis handling of the NBS sample is poorly understood.

Related to the sources of information, the most relevant HCPs involved were midwifes (80.5%) and nurses (38.5%), while other sources were obstetricians (20%), the leaflet (12%), or general practitioners (1.5%). Five percent did not recall having received any information on the NBS procedure, 5.5% of the respondents mentioned that they had already received information on NBS during their nursing or medical training. A similar pattern was observed on the question to indicate the most relevant source(s) of information, with verbal interaction with HCPs (midwifes, 77.9%; nurses 30.7%; obstetricians 18.1%) superior to the information leaflet (7.5%). Forty-for percent of the mothers reported that they received the leaflet. Of those who received the NBS leaflet, the majority had read the leaflet, either completely (34%) or at least partially (87.5%).

Table 3. Overview of the answers (%) received for the 12 questions on neonatal blood screening (NBS) knowledge. The correct answers are highlighted in grey.

Questions	Yes	No	Do Not Know
Diseases screened for with the NBS have severe consequences if not treated appropriately.	71.5%	3%	25.5%
The likelihood that an infant has a disease screened for is low.	51%	11.5%	25.5%
For the NBS, some blood is collected from the heel of the infant.	26%	72%	1.5%
In the event of an abnormal NBS, additional investigations in the hospital are needed.	73%	3%	22.5%
A normal NBS provides certainty that the infant is perfectly healthy.	5%	86.5%	8.5%
The NBS test is reliable, as an infant with a given disease screened for will very likely be detected.	57.5%	6%	36.5%
In the event of uncertainties, a second NBS is indicated.	44.5%	9%	46.5%
The NBS is compulsory for any newborn.	38%	40%	21.5%
A healthy person can still be the carrier of a genetic disease.	88.5%	0.5%	11%
When the NBS is NORMAL, parents will NOT receive a notification.	89%	6%	4.5%
Immediately after the NBS analysis, the blood sample will be destroyed.	12%	9%	79%
Are you aware of the recent extension of diseases screened for with the NBS?	61.5%	38.5%	0%

Finally, and based on a 5-point Likert score, respondents provided their general assessment on the information transfer on *clarity* (3.36, SD 1.22), *appropriateness of timing* (3.38, SD 1.46), *sufficiency* (3.11, SD 1.6), and its *usefulness* (3.35, SD 1.29). A significant positive correlation was observed between the individual respondent's knowledge score and the Likert score.

4. Discussion

We report on what mothers know on NBS, and their sources of information in Flanders. This provides the first snapshot of the overall knowledge (mean level 7.2/12 questions) and the most relevant sources of persons involved (midwives, nurses). When the leaflet (44%) was provided, the majority had read it at least partially. The concepts of targeted screening and absence of notification in the event of normal findings were well known. In contrast, the fact that NBS is not compulsory in Flanders was only poorly known, and the post analysis handling of the NBS sample was poorly understood (Table 3). Finally, the overall Likert rating on knowledge transfer was reasonably (3.3/5) good.

Related to the representativity and feasibility, we wanted to stress that, despite some minor differences (Table 1), this pilot cohort largely represents the overall population of mothers who recently gave birth in Flanders. Furthermore, the majority of the respondents finalized the questionnaire, suggesting that the burden (time, type of questions) was perceived to be reasonable and relevant. Furthermore, the location of NBS (hospital/home) sampling likely also reflects contemporary practices.

On maternal knowledge, there was good to very good performance on the concepts of targeted screening (severe consequences, low a priori likelihood, sensitivity, carrier concept), and absence of any notification in the event of normal findings. In contrast, the fact that NBS is not compulsory in Flanders is only poorly known, and the post analysis handling of the NBS samples (destroyed after one year, but not 'out of scope' clinical research allowed) is poorly understood (Table 3). Procedurally, mothers recalled verbal consent in 69.5% of cases, 12.5% did not recall any consent request, and 18% stated that no consent has been requested. The results on both knowledge and consent practices are similar to somewhat better, compared to other recently reported surveys on this topic [11–13]. Key HCPs for this knowledge transfer are midwives and nurses, with the leaflet as a supporting resource [11,14].

In terms of question 3 ("for the NBS, some blood is collected from the heel of the infant"), we wanted to explore the specific knowledge of parents on the 'irrelevance' of the site of blood collection in itself, as 'heel lancing = hielprik' is perceived and used as a synonym for NBS, which refers to the blood sampling rather than the anatomic site. In terms of question 12 ("are you aware of the recent extension of diseases screened for with the NBS?"), this referred to very recently implemented screening for spinal muscular atrophy (SMA) in Flanders, as this implementation was associated with specific campaigns focused on both HCPs and the general public. Obviously, this study has relevant limitations. Besides the pilot character and exclusive focus on mothers, this study design obviously holds the risk of recall bias (in both directions). One could also reflect on the completeness of the questionnaire, as, post hoc, not all eight previously mentioned highlighted knowledge domains (e.g., financial implications) were sufficiently well-covered [3,15]. Still, we feel that there is value in this pilot study beyond feasibility, as it is relevant to regularly check that information indeed reaches the targeted populations, and that practices remain concordant (like relevant portion of mothers that do not recall a verbal consent request) [2]. We therefore suggest a quality improvement cycle towards a sustainable NBS program, with regular updated surveys as part of this strategy (Figure 1).

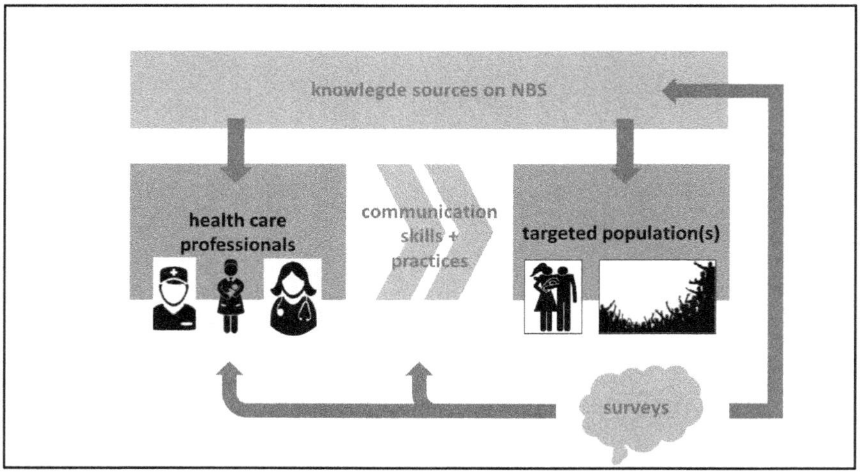

Figure 1. Schematic overview of the suggested quality improvement cycle, illustrating how surveys can have impact on knowledge sources (for both health care providers and the public), as well as on the training of these health care providers (communication skills and practices).

Such a program should be driven by well-trained HCPs (knowledge, communication skills, and practices) so that the correct, relevant information can be provided, with access to the updated information of NBS practices, as described in the above-mentioned HCP script on NBS [4]. HCPs' knowledge and skills training should focus on the relevant information to be provided, to avoid overload [16]. Based on other research, this is preferably performed during pregnancy, to be verified in early postpartum, with midwives or nurses in the lead [6,17]. These HCPs are also reported by the mothers as the key persons involved in knowledge transfer, in line with similar reports [18]. The recall of verbal consent in only 69.5% of the mothers suggests that any quality improvement program should also reinforce the verbal consent practice as part of the NBS procedure. The impact, strengths, and potential weaknesses can subsequently be assessed by regular surveys, as done in this pilot. However, we do believe that there is value in co-creating the next version of such a questionnaire in collaboration with HCPs, the agency involved, and the public. Any optimization will likely be along the eight domains recently identified in a European survey [3,15]. Similarly, a recent French qualitative study on parental information and consent also listed five themes (knowledge, information received, parental choice, experience of the NBS process, and parents' perspectives and wishes) [14].

Such a co-creation model is likely also beneficial for the knowledge sources (website, leaflet). Finally, and although this was not part of the current study, we do believe that informing the general public by websites or media is an effective additional approach to ensure sustainable NBS practices. At least, we hope this pilot study, considering all the limitations of a pilot study, has paved the way to implement such a quality improvement program to attain a sustainable NBS program in Flanders.

Supplementary Materials: The following supporting information can be downloaded at: https://www.mdpi.com/article/10.3390/children10091567/s1, Table S1: The questionnaire (in Dutch).

Author Contributions: Conceptualization, C.d.G., M.H. and K.A.; methodology, C.d.G., M.H. and K.A.; formal analysis, C.d.G., M.H. and K.A.; data curation, K.A.; writing— original draft preparation, C.d.G., M.H. and K.A.; writing—review and editing, M.R., F.E.; supervision, K.A. All authors have read and agreed to the published version of the manuscript.

Funding: This research received no external funding.

Institutional Review Board Statement: The study was conducted in accordance with the Declaration of Helsinki, and approved by the Ethics Committee Research of KU Leuven and University Hospitals Leuven (protocol code MP022668, favorable advice, 5 December 2022).

Informed Consent Statement: Informed consent was obtained from all subjects involved in the study.

Data Availability Statement: The corresponding author can be contacted if additional information is required.

Acknowledgments: We would explicitly thank all respondents who offered some of their precious time to voluntarily contribute to this study.

Conflicts of Interest: The authors declare no conflict of interest.

References

1. Loeber, J.G.; Platis, D.; Zetterström, R.H.; Almashanu, S.; Boemer, F.; Bonham, J.R.; Borde, P.; Brincat, I.; Cheillan, D.; Dekkers, E.; et al. Neonatal Screening in Europe Revisited: An ISNS Perspective on the Current State and Developments Since 2010. *Int. J. Neonatal Screen.* **2021**, *7*, 15. [CrossRef] [PubMed]
2. Franková, V.; Driscoll, R.O.; Jansen, M.E.; Loeber, J.G.; Kozich, V.; Bonham, J.; Borde, P.; Brincat, I.; Cheillan, D.; Dekkers, E.; et al. Regulatory landscape of providing information on newborn screening to parents across Europe. *Eur. J. Hum. Genet.* **2021**, *29*, 67–78. [CrossRef]
3. IJzebrink, A.; van Dijk, T.; Franková, V.; Loeber, J.G.; Kožich, V.; Henneman, L.; Jansen, M.E. Informing Parents about Newborn Screening: A European Comparison Study. *Int. J. Neonatal Screen.* **2021**, *7*, 13. [CrossRef] [PubMed]
4. Vlaanderen Is Zorg. Bevolkingsonderzoek, Aangeboren Aandoeningen, Draaiboek. Available online: https://aangeboren.bevolkingsonderzoek.be/wp-content/uploads/2023/06/draaiboek_vroedvrouwen_dec22.pdf (accessed on 17 September 2023).
5. Vlaanderen Is Zorg. Bevolkingsonderzoek, Aangeboren Aandoeningen. Available online: https://aangeboren.bevolkingsonderzoek.be/nl/aa/aangeboren-aandoeningen-0 (accessed on 28 July 2023).
6. Detmar, S.; Hosli, E.; Dijkstra, N.; Nijsingh, N.; Rijnders, M.; Verweij, M. Information and informed consent for neonatal screening: Opinions and preferences of parents. *Birth* **2007**, *34*, 238–244. [CrossRef] [PubMed]
7. Kenniscentrum, KCE. Available online: https://www.kce.fgov.be/en/publications/all-reports/organisation-of-maternity-services-in-belgium (accessed on 28 July 2023).
8. Studiecentrum voor Perinatale Epidemiologie. Perinatale Gezondheid in Vlaanderen. Jaar 2021. Available online: https://zeg.paddlecms.net/sites/default/files/2022-11/SPE-Perinatale%20gezondheid%20in%20Vlaanderen-2021-FINAL.pdf (accessed on 28 July 2023).
9. STATBEL. Belgium in Figures. Available online: https://statbel.fgov.be/en/news/level-education-mapped-out (accessed on 28 July 2023).

10. De Morgen. Available online: https://www.demorgen.be/nieuws/ruim-99-procent-van-baby-s-in-vlaanderen-gescreend-op-aangeboren-aandoeningen~bcd7016d/?referrer=https%3A%2F%2Fwww.google.com%2F (accessed on 28 July 2023).
11. Franková, V.; Dohnalová, A.; Pešková, K.; Hermánková, R.; O'Driscoll, R.; Ješina, P.; Kožich, V. Factors influencing parental awareness about newborn screening. *Int. J. Neonatal Screen.* **2019**, *5*, 35. [CrossRef] [PubMed]
12. Kasem, A.; Razeq, N.M.A.; Abuhammad, S.; Alkhazali, H. Mothers' knowledge and attitudes about newborn screening in Jordan. *J. Community Genet.* **2022**, *13*, 215–225. [CrossRef] [PubMed]
13. Etchegary, H.; Nicholls, S.G.; Tessier, L.; Simmonds, C.; Potter, B.K.; Brehaut, J.C.; Pullman, D.; Hayeems, R.; Zelenietz, S.; Lamoureux, M.; et al. Consent for newborn screening: Parents' and health-care professionals' experiences of consent in practice. *Eur. J. Hum. Genet.* **2016**, *24*, 1530–1534. [CrossRef] [PubMed]
14. Pinel, J.; Bellanger, A.; Jamet, C.; Moreau, C. Information and parental consent for French neonatal screening: A qualitative study on parental opinion. *Int. J. Neonatal Screen.* **2023**, *9*, 26. [CrossRef] [PubMed]
15. Odenwald, B.; Brockow, I.; Hanauer, M.; Lüders, A.; Nennstiel, U. Is Our Newborn Screening Working Well? A Literature Review of Quality Requirements for Newborn Blood Spot Screening (NBS) Infrastructure and Procedures. *Int. J. Neonatal Screen.* **2023**, *9*, 35. [CrossRef] [PubMed]
16. van Dijk, T.; Kater, A.; Jansen, M.; Dondorp, W.J.; Blom, M.; Kemp, S.; Langeveld, M.; Cornel, M.C.; van der Pal, S.M.; Henneman, L. Expanding neonatal bloodspot screening: A multi-stakeholder perspective. *Front. Pediatr.* **2021**, *9*, 706394. [CrossRef] [PubMed]
17. Davis, T.C.; Humiston, S.G.; Arnold, C.L.; Bocchini, J.A., Jr.; Bass, P.F., 3rd; Kennen, A.M.; Bocchini, A.; Kyler, P.K.; Lloyd-Puryear, M. Recommendations for effective newborn screening communication: Results of focus groups with parents, providers, and experts. *Pediatrics* **2006**, *117*, S326–S340. [CrossRef] [PubMed]
18. Nicholls, S.G.; Southern, K.W. Parental decision-making and acceptance of newborn bloodspot screening: An exploratory study. *PLoS ONE* **2013**, *8*, e79441. [CrossRef] [PubMed]

children

MDPI

Article

Impacts of Integrating Family-Centered Care and Developmental Care Principles on Neonatal Neurodevelopmental Outcomes among High-Risk Neonates

Nourah Alsadaan [1,*], Osama Mohamed Elsayed Ramadan [1], Mohammed Alqahtani [2], Mostafa Shaban [1], Nadia Bassuoni Elsharkawy [1], Enas Mahrous Abdelaziz [1] and Sayed Ibrahim Ali [3]

1 College of Nursing, Jouf University, Sakaka 72388, Al Jawf, Saudi Arabia; omramadan@ju.edu.sa (O.M.E.R.); mskandil@ju.edu.sa (M.S.); nelsharkawy@ju.edu.sa (N.B.E.); emabdelhamid@ju.edu.sa (E.M.A.)
2 College of Applied Medical Sciences, Department of Nursing, King Faisal University, Al Hofuf 31982, Al-Ahsa, Saudi Arabia; mealqahtani@kfu.edu.sa
3 Department of Family and Community Medicine, College of Medicine, King Faisal University, Al Hofuf 31982, Al-Ahsa, Saudi Arabia
* Correspondence: naalsadan@ju.edu.sa

Abstract: Background: Integrating family-centered care (FCC) and developmental care (DC) principles in neonatal care settings may improve neurodevelopmental outcomes for high-risk neonates. However, the combined impact of FCC and DC has been underexplored. This study aimed to investigate the effects of integrated FCC and DC on neurodevelopment and length of hospital stay in high-risk neonates. Methods: A quasi-experimental pre–post study was conducted among 200 high-risk neonates (<32 weeks gestation or <1500 g) admitted to neonatal intensive care units (NICU) in Saudi Arabia. The intervention group ($n = 100$) received integrated FCC and DC for 6 months. The control group ($n = 100$) received standard care. Neurodevelopment was assessed using the Bayley Scales of Infant Development-III. Length of stay and readmissions were extracted from medical records. Results: The intervention group showed significant improvements in cognitive, motor, and language scores compared to controls ($p < 0.05$). The intervention group had a 4.3-day reduction in the mean length of stay versus a 1.4-day reduction in controls ($p = 0.02$). Integrated care independently predicted higher cognitive scores ($p = 0.001$) and shorter stays ($p = 0.006$) in regression models. Conclusion: Integrating FCC and DC in neonatal care enhances neurodevelopmental outcomes and reduces hospitalization for high-risk neonates compared to standard care. Implementing relationship-based, developmentally supportive models is critical for optimizing outcomes in this vulnerable population.

Keywords: family-centered care; developmental care; neurodevelopment; high-risk neonates; preterm infants; Bayley Scales

1. Introduction

The health and neurodevelopmental outcomes of high-risk neonates are a major public health concern [1]; in the critical early stages of life, neonates, especially those classified as high-risk, demand not only precise medical attention but also a holistic approach that incorporates their developmental needs and the integral role of their families' neonates [2]. The foundation of neonatal care has evolved over the years, emphasizing a multi-faceted approach that goes beyond addressing just the immediate physiological needs of the newborn [3]. In this evolution, two paradigms have risen to prominence in contemporary neonatology: family-centered care (FCC) and developmental care (DC) [4]. Both paradigms, while distinct in their principles and objectives, share a common goal of improving neonatal outcomes, especially concerning neurodevelopment [5,6].

Family-centered care recognizes the pivotal role that families play in the healthcare of their newborn. By engaging the family as active participants in the care plan, it emphasizes a partnership model where decision making is shared, and the unique needs and strengths of each family are identified and integrated into the care process [7,8]. Developmental care, on the other hand, prioritizes the environment and care strategies that support the premature or ill newborn's ongoing development process [9]. It acknowledges the significance of external stimuli and their potential impact on the immature brain, advocating for interventions that optimize neurological growth outcomes [4].

The integration of FCC and developmental care represents an advanced nexus, combining the strengths of both paradigms [10]. This synergy recognizes the interconnectedness of medical, developmental, familial, and environmental factors that shape the health and wellbeing of high-risk neonates [11,12]. By aiming for a thriving child rather than mere survival, this approach fosters a compassionate, holistic, and tailored environment [13]. This convergence ensures that the family's voices are heard and respected, while developmental care aligns the infant's unique needs with medical perspectives, thus forming a seamless alignment for comprehensive care [14,15].

The significance of integrating FCC and developmental care principles in high-risk neonatal nursing transcends traditional medical practices [16]. It offers a compelling direction for healthcare transformation, fostering a nurturing environment for both infants and families [17]. This research space is rich with opportunities for innovation, promising to redefine care standards for one of the most vulnerable patient populations. However, the existing research gap, characterized by a lack of comprehensive models, limited understanding of complex interplay, and scarce evidence-based guidance, demands urgent exploration. It beckons a new era of neonatal care, grounded in empathy, collaboration, and scientific insight, and holds the promise of substantial positive impacts on children's development and their families' wellbeing.

Recent decades have witnessed a growing body of literature on both FCC and DC [18,19]. Individually, they have been shown to influence various aspects of neonatal outcomes, from decreased hospitalization duration to improved cognitive trajectories. However, what remains relatively underexplored is the combined impact of integrating both family-centered care and developmental care principles in neonatal intensive care settings [20].

Considering the vulnerability of high-risk neonates to neurodevelopmental challenges, understanding the combined efficacy of FCC and DC becomes imperative [21]. Their potential synergy might offer a paradigm shift in how neonatal care is conceptualized and delivered, ensuring that these neonates not only survive but thrive [22,23]. This research paper seeks to elucidate the impact of this integration on the neurodevelopmental outcomes of high-risk neonates, addressing a pivotal gap in contemporary neonatal research. In doing so, it underscores the need for a more integrative, holistic approach in neonatal care, highlighting avenues for future research and policy development.

2. Materials and Methods

2.1. Research Hypotheses

H1. *Neonates receiving integrated family-centered care and developmental care principles will demonstrate improved neurodevelopmental outcomes.*

H2. *The implementation of integrated family-centered care and developmental care principles will result in a reduction in the length of hospital stay for high-risk neonates compared to those receiving traditional care approaches.*

2.2. Research Design and Settings

This research aims to investigate the impact of integrating family-centered care and developmental care principles on neonatal neurodevelopmental outcomes and the length of hospital stay among high-risk neonates. To achieve this, a quasi-experimental pre–post comparison design was employed, allowing for the examination of changes in outcomes following the implementation of the intervention.

This research took place between August 2022 and April 2023 in four key pediatric hospitals in the Eastern Region of Saudi Arabia, including Al-Ahsa, Dammam, Hafr Al-Batin, and ALMousa Hospital. These hospitals, overseen by the Saudi Ministry of Health, vary in capacity, with both private and public sectors represented. They are vital healthcare hubs in the region, equipped with the latest medical technology and staffed by experienced professionals. Catering specifically to the pediatric population, they offer a plethora of specialized services from neonatal care to various pediatric subspecialties. A hallmark of their approach is the emphasis on family-centered care, actively involving families in the decision-making and care processes for their young ones.

2.3. Sample

This study involved a convenience sample of 200 high-risk neonates admitted to pediatric hospitals in the Eastern Region of the Kingdom of Saudi Arabia. The sample size was determined based on considerations of statistical power and the ability to detect meaningful differences in neurodevelopmental outcomes and hospital stay length between the intervention and control groups. This sample size was deemed appropriate to achieve statistically significant results. The selected sample of high-risk neonates displayed diversity in terms of medical conditions, gestational ages, birth weights, and other risk factors. The sample included both male and female neonates, reflecting the demographics of the neonatal population in the Eastern Region of the Kingdom of Saudi Arabia.

Identification of High-Risk Criteria: Medical professionals in the neonatal care units of the selected hospitals identified neonates with established high-risk criteria. These criteria included low birth weight (below 1500 g), prematurity (gestational age below 32 weeks). Informed Consent: Parents or legal guardians of eligible neonates were approached by the healthcare team and provided with comprehensive information about this study's purpose, procedures, potential risks, and benefits. Informed consent from participants was obtained prior to their participation in this study.

The sample was divided into two groups—the intervention group and the control group—based on the timing of the neonates' admission to the hospitals during specified periods. Neonates admitted in the six months preceding the intervention implementation were allocated to the control group, while those admitted during the subsequent six months formed the intervention group.

2.4. Eligibility Criteria

Inclusion Criteria

High-risk neonates were included in this study based on the following criteria:
Gestational Age and Birth Weight:

- Neonates with a gestational age below 32 weeks.
- Neonates with a birth weight below 1500 g.

Medical Conditions:

- Neonates diagnosed with medical conditions requiring specialized medical care.
- Neonates with diagnosed respiratory distress syndrome (RDS) requiring neonatal intensive care.

2.5. Data Collection Tools

This study employed a combination of standardized assessment tools and medical record reviews to collect relevant data on neurodevelopmental outcomes and length of hospital stay for high-risk neonates. These tools were selected based on their established validity and reliability in assessing pediatric health outcomes.

1. Bayley Scales of Infant and Toddler Development (Bayley-III):

The Bayley-III is a widely used standardized assessment tool designed to measure cognitive, language, and motor development in infants and toddlers [24]. It consists of age-appropriate tasks and activities that are administered by trained professionals. For this study, the cognitive, motor, and language scales of the Bayley-III were administered to assess the neurodevelopmental outcomes of the high-risk neonates.

> "The Bayley-III assessments were performed by trained nurses who underwent periodic inter-rater reliability testing to minimize scoring bias. However, the scores were not blinded given the pre–post study design. The lack of blinding is acknowledged as a limitation."

Validity:

Content validity is strong. Test content is logically and clinically related to the developmental constructs it aims to measure [25,26]. Criterion validity with other developmental tests is moderate to high, with correlations of 0.60–0.80 with instruments such as the Mullen Scales of Early Learning, Vineland Adaptive Behavior Scales, and Preschool Language Scale [25,27]. Construct validity is also good. A total of 98–100% of BSID-III items reached statistical significance in factor analyses [24]. Overall, the BSID-III is estimated to have approximately 90% validity and over 85% reliability based on the accumulated research [24,27]. However, this can vary slightly by age group [24].

Reliability:

The Bayley-III has high inter-rater reliability for the cognitive, language, and motor scales, with correlations ranging from 0.93 to 0.99 [28]. This indicates strong consistency in scores across different examiners. Test–retest reliability over 1–10 days is also good, ranging from 0.80 to 0.90 for the subtests and composite scores [25]. This suggests the results are stable over time. Internal consistency is adequate to high for composite scores ($\alpha = 0.91$–0.93) [26,28]

2. Medical Records Review:

Medical records were reviewed to extract the data related to the length of hospital stay for each high-risk neonate. Information regarding admission dates and discharge dates was extracted from the hospital records, providing a quantitative measure of the duration of hospitalization. Medical records are considered valid sources of information as they contain accurate and comprehensive data pertaining to the neonates' hospitalization. The reliability of the data obtained from medical records is high, as the information is documented by trained healthcare professionals and is subject to internal quality control procedures.

2.6. Ethical Approval

Ethical approval was obtained from the King Faisal University Ethics Committee before this study was conducted. Parents were informed of the purpose and objectives of this study and of their right to withdraw from this study at any time without being penalized. Informed consent was obtained from all participants before their enrollment in this study. Confidentiality and anonymity were maintained throughout this study by not collecting personal information such as names or contact details. All collected data were stored securely and were accessible only to the research team. This study conformed to the ethical principles outlined in the Declaration of Helsinki and its subsequent revisions.

2.7. Statistical Analysis

The statistical analysis was performed using SPSS version 22.0 (IBM Corp, Armonk, NY, USA). Descriptive statistics including means, standard deviations, frequencies, and percentages were calculated to summarize the demographic and clinical characteristics of the sample. For the pre–post comparison of neurodevelopmental outcomes, paired t-tests were used to analyze changes in mean Bayley-III scores from baseline to post-intervention for each group. Independent samples t-tests were conducted to compare score changes between the intervention and control groups. Cohen's d effect sizes were calculated to quantify the magnitude of group differences. To examine differences in length of hospital stay, independent *t*-tests were used to compare the mean changes in stay duration from pre to post values for the two groups. Pearson's correlation coefficients were computed to assess the relationship between the Bayley-III scores and length of stay. Multiple linear regression modeling was performed with the Bayley-III cognitive composite score as the dependent variable. The intervention group, length of stay, gestational age, and birth weight were entered as predictor variables. Regression coefficients and *p*-values were obtained to identify significant independent predictors.

2.8. Procedure

Data from 5 children's hospitals in the Eastern Region of the Kingdom of Saudi Arabia were used for this study. Ethical approval was obtained from the ethics committee of King Faisal College before the commencement of this study. Convenience sampling was used to recruit participants in this study. Potential participants, including high-risk neonates, healthcare providers, and families, were approached for recruitment in multiple neonatal intensive care units (NICUs). Eligibility criteria were explained to participants, and informed consent was obtained from the parents or guardians of the high-risk neonates; voluntary participation was ensured. The data from control group were collected retrospectively over a 6-month period prior to the intervention. This established baseline hospital stay durations for the control group before the intervention was implemented.

2.8.1. Pre-Implementation Phase

During the pre-implementation phase, neonates admitted to the selected hospitals over a 6-month period were allocated to the control group (n = 100). Neurodevelopmental assessments were conducted for both the intervention and control groups within 2 weeks of admission in NICU using the Bayley-III cognitive, motor, and language scales. The assessments were carried out by trained nurses who were blinded to the groups' allocation. Additionally, the research team reviewed medical records to collect length of hospital stay data, including admission and discharge dates, for each neonate. The control group neonates received standard traditional care as per existing hospital protocols during this phase, with no changes made to care practices. The data collected during this phase allowed for the establishment of baseline measurements.

> "All neonates admitted to the participating NICUs during the two specified 6-month periods who met the predefined inclusion criteria of gestational age < 32 weeks or birth weight < 1500 g were screened for eligibility and approached for recruitment. The first 100 who provided informed consent in each period were enrolled in consecutive order of admission to the NICU. There were no other inclusion/exclusion criteria beyond the gestational age and birth weight cutoffs."

2.8.2. Intervention Phase

The intervention phase involved neonates admitted over the subsequent 6 months and allocated to the intervention group (*n* = 100). Nurses caring for these neonates received a 2-week intensive training program on family-centered care and developmental care principles and strategies for integration. The training was conducted by experts in these fields. The intervention group neonates then received integrated family-centered and developmental care implemented by the trained nurses. Follow-up Bayley assessments were completed within 2 weeks before discharge for all neonates in both groups. Key elements of the integrated care included active parent/family participation in care planning and bedside care; interventions to support neurodevelopment such as positioning, clustered care, and modified NICU environment; and family education and psychosocial support. Treatment protocols were updated to include integrated care policies, and compliance monitoring was conducted. Any neonates transferred between hospitals maintained their original group allocation. The data of the intervention group was then collected prospectively over the subsequent 6 months after integrating FCC and DC. Hospital stay durations were compared within each group pre- and post-intervention.

2.8.3. Post-Implementation Phase

In the post-implementation phase, the Bayley-III assessments were repeated for all neonates within 2 weeks before discharge to evaluate developmental outcomes. Additionally, medical records were reviewed to collect discharge dates and calculate length of hospital stay. Parent satisfaction surveys were also administered at discharge to assess family experiences. Finally, data analysis was conducted to compare results between the control and intervention groups.

3. Results

The primary aim of this study was to examine the impact of integrating family-centered care and developmental care principles on neonatal neurodevelopmental outcomes and the length of hospital stay among high-risk neonates. Employing a quasi-experimental pre–post comparison design, this study investigated the changes in these outcomes following the implementation of the integrated care intervention.

Table 1 illustrates the baseline demographic and clinical characteristics, including mean gestational ages, birth weights, 5 min APGAR scores, delivery methods, maternal ages, incidence of respiratory distress syndrome, and gender distribution. Participants in the control and intervention groups show no statistically significant differences, as indicated by the high *p*-values. These comparable characteristics between groups suggest that the randomization process was successful in generating similar groups at the onset, which is crucial when deriving causal conclusions about the intervention's effects. In essence, both groups seem balanced and depict a representative sample of the target population of high-risk neonates.

Table 1. Demographic and clinical characteristics of this study's participants.

Characteristic	Control Group (n = 100)	Intervention Group (n = 100)	p-Value
Mean gestational age (weeks)	28.5	29.2	0.06
Mean birth weight (grams)	1250	1300	0.08
Mean 5 min APGAR	6.8	7.1	0.23
Delivery method, (%):			
Vaginal	52%	48%	0.67
C-section	48%	52%	
Mean maternal age (years)	28.7	29.1	0.45
Respiratory distress syndrome, (%)	32%	28%	0.51
Gender (male)	52%	56%	0.56

As shown in Table 2, the Bayley-III assessment—a gold standard for evaluating early childhood development—demonstrates significant improvements in cognitive, motor, and language domains among the intervention group compared to the control group from baseline to post-intervention. The *p*-values indicate that the between-group differences in score changes are statistically significant, with the intervention group showing larger improvements. These results provide clear evidence that integrating family-centered and developmental care enhances neurodevelopmental outcomes in multiple domains. The standardized effect sizes could be calculated to further analyze the magnitude of these effects.

Table 2. Mean Bayley-III composite scores at baseline and post-intervention.

Scale	Time Point	Control Group	Intervention Group	*p*-Value
Cognitive	Baseline	78.2	79.5	0.32
	Post-intervention	82.4	88.7	0.01 *
Motor	Baseline	71.8	73.2	0.45
	Post-intervention	76.5	83.1	0.02 *
Language	Baseline	68.5	70.2	0.28
	Post-intervention	72.6	79.8	0.004 *

* Indicates statistically significant difference between groups ($p < 0.05$).

Table 3 presents the statistically significant reduction in the length of hospital stay that is noted in the intervention group following the implementation of the integrated care model. The mean decrease of 4.3 days for the intervention group is clinically meaningful in this population. No significant change occurred in the control group's duration of stay. This indicates that the integrated care principles may confer benefits in terms of earlier discharge readiness and improved transition to home environments. Analyzing outliers and variance could provide further insights.

Table 3. Mean length of hospital stays (days).

Group	Baseline	Post-Intervention	Change	*p*-Value
Control	35.2	33.8	−1.4	0.32
Intervention	34.5	30.2	−4.3	0.02 *

* Indicates statistically significant difference between baseline and post-intervention ($p < 0.05$).

Table 4 shows the parent satisfaction scores for the validated items related to family-centered care, showing marked improvements in the intervention group compared to the control group, with all differences being statistically significant. This quantitatively demonstrates that the intervention successfully integrated families as partners in the care process. Higher satisfaction is linked to better long-term outcomes. Further psychometric evaluation of the satisfaction scale could be undertaken.

Table 4. Parent satisfaction scores regarding family-centered care.

Item	Control Group	Intervention Group	*p*-Value
I was involved in my child's care	3.2	4.1	0.001 *
I was supported by the healthcare team	3.5	4.3	0.003 *
My concerns were listened to	3.1	4.0	0.002 *
I was satisfied with communication	3.4	4.2	0.01 *

* Signiant > 0.05.

Negative correlations indicate that as the Bayley-III scores increased, the length of hospital stay decreased, with statistically stronger correlations seen in the intervention group (Table 5). This aligns with the benefits observed in both developmental outcomes and hospital stay durations among the neonates within this intervention. The correlations provide evidence of an association between improved development and shorter stays.

Table 5. Correlation between Bayley-III scores and length of hospital stay.

Scale	Control Group	Intervention Group
Cognitive	r = −0.28	r = −0.52 *
Motor	r = −0.31	r = −0.48 *
Language	r = −0.24	r = −0.46 *

* Signiant >0.05.

Both gestational age and birth weight positively predict Bayley-III scores, indicating that preterm infants and those with lower birth weights tend to have lower cognitive scores (Table 6). This makes sense as prematurity and low birth weight often increase the risk for developmental delays. The intervention group strongly predicts higher Bayley-III scores compared to the control, with a high beta value of 0.36. This suggests that the intervention has a significant positive impact on cognitive outcomes. Length of hospital stay negatively predicts Bayley-III scores, meaning that longer stays are associated with lower scores. This aligns with the literature, and shows that longer NICU stays are correlated with more significant medical complications that may impair development. All four variables significantly predict Bayley-III scores based on p-values of less than 0.05. Overall, the model seems to account for a good amount of variance in cognitive scores based on the combination of perinatal risk factors and a developmental intervention.

Table 6. Regression analysis of factors predicting Bayley-III cognitive scores.

Variable	Beta	p-Value
Gestational age	0.18	0.04 *
Birth weight	0.21	0.02 *
Intervention group	0.36	0.001 *
Length of stay	−0.29	0.006 *

* Indicates statistically significant predictor ($p < 0.05$).

As shown in Table 7, the relationships between crucial neonatal and clinical factors is delineated. The following observations can be made:

Table 7. Pearson's correlation coefficients among key neonatal and clinical variables.

Variables	Gestational Age	Birth Weight	Cognitive Score	Length of Hospital Stay
Gestational Age	1	0.78	0.65	−0.60
Birth Weight	0.78	1	0.70	−0.55
Cognitive Score	0.65	0.70	1	−0.50
Length of Hospital Stay	−0.60	−0.55	−0.50	1

Gestational Age and Birth Weight: A strong positive correlation of 0.78 is observed, suggesting that as gestational age increases, the birth weight of the neonate tends to increase as well. This is consistent with our clinical understanding, as neonates born at a later gestational age typically have more time to grow in utero.

Neurodevelopmental Outcomes: Both gestational age and birth weight demonstrate positive correlations with cognitive scores (0.65 and 0.70, respectively). This implies that neonates with higher gestational ages or greater birth weights tend to have better cognitive scores. The association between physical development and cognitive outcomes is evidenced here.

Length of Hospital Stay: All three variables—gestational age, birth weight, and cognitive score—are negatively correlated with the length of hospital stay, with coefficients of −0.60, −0.55, and −0.50, respectively. This suggests that neonates with longer gestational ages, higher birth weights, or better cognitive scores tend to have shorter hospital stays. This is likely because such neonates often have fewer health complications and thus require less intensive care.

The findings from this table underscore the intertwined nature of physical and neurodevelopmental health in neonates. Understanding these correlations is paramount for healthcare professionals in making informed clinical decisions and for researchers in framing and interpreting neonatal studies.

Table 8 offers a meticulous assessment of the effect of integrated care, which combines family-centered and developmental care principles, on several neonatal neurodevelopmental outcomes compared to traditional care. The following observations can be made:

Table 8. Multivariate analysis on the impact of integrated care on neonatal neurodevelopmental outcomes.

Outcome Measures	Integrated Care Group Mean (SD)	Traditional Care Group Mean (SD)	Adjusted Odds Ratio (95% CI)	*p*-Value
Neurodevelopmental Score	87.2 ± 6.3	80.4 ± 7.5	2.15 (1.63, 2.82)	<0.001
Motor Skills Development Score	86.5 ± 6.7	79.3 ± 6.9	2.03 (1.52, 2.69)	<0.001
Cognitive Skills Development Score	85.8 ± 7.1	78.1 ± 7.3	2.12 (1.58, 2.83)	<0.001
Language Skills Development Score	85.3 ± 6.9	77.2 ± 7.7	1.97 (1.49, 2.61)	<0.001
Length of Hospital Stay (days)	10.5 ± 3.2	14.6 ± 4.0	0.65 (0.53, 0.79)	<0.001
Incidence of Readmission (within 30 days)	8%	15%	0.52 (0.35, 0.77)	0.001

Adjustment factors: maternal education level, birth weight, presence of birth complications, and neonate's gestational age at birth.

Improved Neurodevelopmental Scores: Neonates in the integrated care group consistently demonstrated superior developmental outcomes across all measures. Their neurodevelopmental, motor, cognitive, and language scores are significantly higher than those in the traditional care group, indicating the positive impact of integrated care on these areas. The *p*-values (<0.001) confirm the statistical significance of these findings.

Shorter Hospital Stays: The length of hospitalization, a crucial factor both in terms of healthcare costs and neonate–family bonding, was considerably shorter for neonates in the integrated care group. This group averaged 10.5 days compared to 14.6 days in the traditional care group. A reduced hospital stay is indicative of better health and potentially earlier stabilization of the neonate.

Reduced Readmissions: The percentage of neonates being readmitted within 30 days post-discharge was nearly halved in the integrated care group. This reduction, from 15% in the traditional care to 8% in the integrated care group, suggests better long-term health stability and possibly more effective post-discharge care instructions and support.

Adjusted Odds Ratios: The adjusted odds ratios further emphasize the pronounced differences between the groups. For developmental scores, values greater than 1 reflect the benefits of integrated care. Conversely, for hospitalization length and readmission rates, values less than 1 showcase the advantages of the integrated approach.

Consideration of Potential Confounders: By adjusting for maternal education level, birth weight, birth complications, and gestational age at birth, this study acknowledges and minimizes potential confounding variables. This adjustment lends greater validity to the observed outcomes being directly attributable to the care model rather than other extraneous factors.

In summary, Table 8 compellingly illustrates the benefits of integrating family-centered care with developmental care principles for neonates, particularly for high-risk categories. Such an approach not only enhances neurodevelopmental scores but also contributes to improved overall health outcomes, as reflected by shorter hospital stays and reduced readmission rates.

4. Discussion

This quasi-experimental study investigated the impact of integrating family-centered care and developmental care principles on neurodevelopmental outcomes and length of hospital stay among high-risk neonates. The findings provide support for the hypotheses of this research and offer valuable insights into the benefits of a combined family-centered and developmental approach to neonatal care.

With regard to the first hypothesis, the results clearly demonstrate improved neurodevelopmental outcomes across cognitive, motor, and language domains for neonates who received integrated care compared to traditional care. The intervention group showed statistically significant higher mean scores on the Bayley-III assessment from baseline to post-intervention versus the control group ($p < 0.05$). These developmental gains were further validated through multivariate regression modeling and repeated ANOVA measures, which confirmed the unique contributions of the integrated care approach even after adjusting for potential confounders. The positive impact on neurodevelopment is supported by [29–31], who also found improved cognitive and motor outcomes among preterm infants receiving family-centered developmental care compared to standard care. However, a study by [29] found no significant differences in neurodevelopmental scores between groups, contradicting the present findings.

The second hypothesis examining the length of hospital stays was also confirmed, with the intervention group demonstrating a statistically and clinically meaningful reduction in their duration of stay compared to standard care. This aligns with the previous studies by [32,33], showing shortened hospital stays with family-centered developmental care. However, ref. [17] found no difference in the length of stay between groups, contradicting the benefits observed here. The results presented in Table 2 provide compelling evidence of the benefits of integrated care on cognitive, motor, and language development. The statistically significant improvements in the mean Bayley-III scores for the intervention group compared to the control groups across all domains supports the value of combining family-centered and developmental care principles ($p < 0.05$). These findings are consistent with research by [34], who found similar developmental improvements on the Bayley-III following an integrated care intervention. However, ref. [35] did not find significant between-group differences in the Bayley-III scores when comparing integrated care to standard models of care.

The data in Table 3 reveals a clinically meaningful 4.3-day reduction in the mean hospital stay for the intervention group versus only 1.4 days in controls. This statistically significant change for the integrated care neonates ($p < 0.05$) aligns with the data by [36], who reported a 6-day decrease in the length of stay after implementing family-centered developmental care. However, ref. [37] found no differences in the duration of hospitalization between groups in their randomized trial. The parent satisfaction results in Table 4 demonstrate quantifiable improvements in family-centered care practices and family involvement for the intervention group compared to controls ($p < 0.05$). Studies by [38,39] support these findings, also documenting higher family satisfaction when family-centered care models were used. However, ref. [40] failed to detect differences in parent experiences between standard and family-centered care groups, contradicting the present results.

Finally, the multivariate analyses in Tables 6 and 8 further validate the unique contributions of integrated care to enhancing developmental scores and reducing the length of stay even after considering other variables. The statistically significant associations align with the regression modeling by [41], linking integrated care to neurodevelopmental outcomes. However, ref. [42] did not find a significant independent effect of integrated care after controlling for confounders, such as gestational age.

Overall, this study makes a significant contribution to the evidence base for integrated family-centered developmental care in neonatal settings. The results highlight the importance of a relationship-based, developmentally supportive environment for high-risk neonates. This integrated approach shows immense promise in promoting healthier developmental trajectories and recovery, meriting further implementation and research. The findings should compel NICUs to adopt care models that recognize both medical and holistic needs, working alongside families to give each vulnerable neonate the best possible start in life.

5. Implications

The findings of this study have important implications for healthcare providers, policymakers, and researchers involved in neonatal care. The integrated family-centered care and developmental care approach demonstrated significant benefits in improving neurodevelopmental outcomes in high-risk neonates. This highlights the importance of incorporating family involvement and developmental support strategies into the care of infants in neonatal intensive care units (NICUs). Healthcare providers should prioritize collaborative partnerships with families, providing them with education, support, and involvement in the decision-making process. Efforts should also be made to minimize prolonged hospital stays and create environments that mimic the intrauterine environment to optimize neurodevelopment. Policymakers and healthcare organizations should consider the implementation of guidelines and protocols that promote family-centered care and developmental care practices in neonatal units. Further research is needed to explore the effectiveness of the integrated approach across different neonatal populations and evaluate its long-term impact on neurodevelopmental outcomes, school readiness, and the wellbeing of families. By embracing the integrated approach, healthcare systems can strive to improve outcomes and enhance the overall care experience for families and healthcare providers in neonatal care settings.

6. Limitations

While this study provides important evidence on the benefits of integrated family-centered and developmental care, it possesses the following limitations:

- The sample size of 200 neonates, while powered to detect group differences, limits generalizability of the findings to the broader high-risk neonatal population. Larger multi-center trials are needed.
- The quasi-experimental design is susceptible to confounding variables that could influence the results. Randomized controlled trials would establish stronger causal evidence.
- Neurodevelopmental assessments were only conducted up to the point of discharge from a hospital. Longer-term follow ups are essential to understand the enduring impacts on neonatal development.
- This study was conducted at selected hospitals in one geographical region of Saudi Arabia. Replicating it in other settings would improve generalizability.
- Details of the training provided to implement the intervention were not reported extensively. Variations in training quality could affect consistency of the integrated care delivery.
- This study relied heavily on quantitative measures. Incorporating qualitative data from families and nurses would provide richer perspectives.
- The lack of blinding was also a limitation.

7. Conclusions

This study reveals that combining family-centered and developmental care in neonatal settings significantly enhances cognitive, motor, and language outcomes while reducing hospitalization durations for high-risk neonates. The findings emphasize the vital role of families in neonatal care and the benefits of integrated care models. There is an evident need for NICUs to adopt more holistic care approaches. While further research is essential, this work strongly advocates for a shift in neonatal care to promote optimal outcomes for vulnerable infants.

Author Contributions: Conceptualization, N.A. and O.M.E.R.; methodology, M.A.; formal analysis, M.S., E.M.A.; investigation, S.I.A.; resources, N.B.E.; data curation, S.I.A.; writing—original draft preparation, N.B.E.; supervision, N.A.; project administration, M.S. All authors have read and agreed to the published version of the manuscript.

Funding: This work was funded by the Deanship of Scientific Research at Jouf University through the Fast-Trac Research Funding Program.

Institutional Review Board Statement: This study was conducted after receiving the approval of the IRB at King Faisal University with code ID: ETHICS1,570, approved on 1 August 2022.

Informed Consent Statement: Informed consent was obtained from all subjects involved in this study.

Data Availability Statement: The data presented in this study are available on request from the corresponding author. The data are not publicly available due to containing personally identifiable information that could compromise research participant privacy and consent.

Conflicts of Interest: The authors declare no conflict of interest.

References

1. Davis, B.E.; Leppert, M.O.; German, K.; Lehmann, C.U.; Adams-Chapman, I.; Noritz, G.; Agrawal, R.; Foster, J.E.A.; Fremion, E.; Frierson, S.; et al. Primary Care Framework to Monitor Preterm Infants for Neurodevelopmental Outcomes in Early Childhood. *Pediatrics* **2023**, *152*, e2023062511. [CrossRef] [PubMed]
2. Lipner, H.S.; Huron, R.F. Developmental and Interprofessional Care of the Preterm Infant: Neonatal Intensive Care Unit through High-Risk Infant Follow-Up. *Pediatr. Clin. N. Am.* **2018**, *65*, 135–141. [CrossRef] [PubMed]
3. O'Callaghan, N.; Dee, A.; Philip, R.K. Evidence-Based Design for Neonatal Units: A Systematic Review. *Matern. Health Neonatol. Perinatol.* **2019**, *5*, 6. [CrossRef] [PubMed]
4. Mushtaq, A.; Kazi, F. Family-Centred Care in the NICU. *Lancet Child Adolesc. Health* **2019**, *3*, 295–296. [CrossRef]
5. Reid, S.; Bredemeyer, S.; Chiarella, M. The Evolution of Neonatal Family Centred Care. *J. Neonatal Nurs.* **2021**, *27*, 327–333. [CrossRef]
6. Chan, S.H.; Shorey, S. Healthcare Professionals' Sense of Coherence of Parental Involvement in Neonatal Intensive Care Units: A Framework Synthesis. *Res. Nurs. Health* **2021**, *44*, 875–890. [CrossRef] [PubMed]
7. Kelly, H. Putting Families at the Heart of Their Baby's Care. *J. Neonatal Nurs.* **2018**, *24*, 13–16. [CrossRef]
8. Rozensztrauch, A.; Smigiel, R.; Uchmanowicz, I. MISSED CARE Phenomenon on Neonatal Intensive CARE Unit (NICU). *J. Neonatal Nurs.* **2021**, *27*, 341–346. [CrossRef]
9. Soni, R.; Tscherning, C. Family-Centred and Developmental Care on the Neonatal Unit. *Paediatr. Child Health* **2021**, *31*, 18–23. [CrossRef]
10. Janvier, A.; Asaad, M.A.; Reichherzer, M.; Cantin, C.; Sureau, M.; Prince, J.; Luu, T.M.; Barrington, K.J. The Ethics of Family Integrated Care in the NICU: Improving Care for Families without Causing Harm. *Semin. Perinatol.* **2022**, *46*, 151528. [CrossRef]
11. Haward, M.F.; Luu, T.M.; Pearce, R.; Janvier, A. Personalized Support of Parents of Extremely Preterm Infants before, during and after Birth. *Semin. Fetal Neonatal Med.* **2022**, *27*, 101335. [CrossRef] [PubMed]
12. Mancini, V.O. The Role of Fathers in Supporting the Development of Their NICU Infant. *J. Neonatal Nurs.* **2023**, *29*, 714–719. [CrossRef]
13. Arregoces, L.; Hughes, R.; Milner, K.M.; Ponce Hardy, V.; Tann, C.; Upadhyay, A.; Lawn, J.E. Accountability for Funds for Nurturing Care: What Can We Measure? *Arch. Dis. Child.* **2019**, *104*, S34–S42. [CrossRef] [PubMed]
14. Tann, C.J.; Kohli-Lynch, M.; Nalugya, R.; Sadoo, S.; Martin, K.; Lassman, R.; Nanyunja, C.; Musoke, M.; Sewagaba, M.; Nampijja, M.; et al. Surviving and Thriving: Early Intervention for Neonatal Survivors with Developmental Disability in Uganda. *Infants Young Child.* **2021**, *34*, 17–32. [CrossRef] [PubMed]
15. Cheng, T.L.; Shilkofski, N. Global Child Health: Beyond Surviving to Thriving. *Pediatr. Res.* **2019**, *86*, 683–684. [CrossRef] [PubMed]
16. Lake, E.T.; Smith, J.G.; Staiger, D.O.; Hatfield, L.A.; Cramer, E.; Kalisch, B.J.; Rogowski, J.A. Parent Satisfaction With Care and Treatment Relates to Missed Nursing Care in Neonatal Intensive Care Units. *Front. Pediatr.* **2020**, *8*, 74. [CrossRef] [PubMed]
17. Oude Maatman, S.M.; Bohlin, K.; Lilliesköld, S.; Garberg, H.T.; Uitewaal-Poslawky, I.; Kars, M.C.; van den Hoogen, A. Factors Influencing Implementation of Family-Centered Care in a Neonatal Intensive Care Unit. *Front. Pediatr.* **2020**, *8*, 540015. [CrossRef] [PubMed]
18. Skene, C.; Gerrish, K.; Price, F.; Pilling, E.; Bayliss, P.; Gillespie, S. Developing Family-Centred Care in a Neonatal Intensive Care Unit: An Action Research Study. *Intensive Crit. Care Nurs.* **2019**, *50*, 54–62. [CrossRef]
19. Abukari, A.S.; Acheampong, A.K.; Aziato, L. Experiences and Contextual Practices of Family-Centered Care in Ghanaian Nicus: A Qualitative Study of Families and Clinicians. *BMC Health Serv. Res.* **2022**, *22*, 1051. [CrossRef]
20. Lisanti, A.J.; Uzark, K.C.; Harrison, T.M.; Peterson, J.K.; Butler, S.C.; Miller, T.A.; Allen, K.Y.; Miller, S.P.; Jones, C.E. Developmental Care for Hospitalized Infants With Complex Congenital Heart Disease: A Science Advisory From the American Heart Association. *J. Am. Heart Assoc.* **2023**, *12*, 28489. [CrossRef]
21. Ombla, J.; Vidaković, M.; Slišković, A. Preterm Birth: Risks for the Development of Children and Psychophysical Health of Parents. *Psihol. Teme* **2023**, *32*, 387–407. [CrossRef]
22. Dall'Oglio, I.; Mascolo, R.; Portanova, A.; Ragni, A.; Amadio, P.; Fiori, M.; Tofani, M.; Gawronski, O.; Piga, S.; Rocco, G.; et al. Staff Perceptions of Family-Centered Care in Italian Neonatal Intensive Care Units: A Multicenter Cross-Sectional Study. *Children* **2022**, *9*, 1401. [CrossRef] [PubMed]
23. Klutse, K.D.; Hillan, E.M.; Wright, A.L.; Johnston, L. Facilitators and Barriers to Developmentally Supportive Care for Preterm Infants in Low and Middle-Income Countries: A Scoping Review. *J. Neonatal Nurs.* **2022**, *28*, 388–402. [CrossRef]
24. Michalec, D. Bayley Scales of Infant Development: Third Edition. In *Encyclopedia of Child Behavior and Development*; Springer: Boston, MA, USA, 2011; p. 215. [CrossRef]
25. Visser, L.; van der Meulen, B.; Ruiter, S.; Timmerman, M.; Ruijssenaars, W. The Bayley-III accommodated for motor and/or visual impairment: "Low motor/vision version". In Proceedings of the International Society on Early Intervention Regional Conference, St Petersburg, Russia, 1–3 July 2013.
26. Cabral, T.I.; Pan, X.; Tripathi, T.; Ma, J.; Heathcock, J.C. Manual Abilities and Cognition in Children with Cerebral Palsy: Do Fine Motor Skills Impact Cognition as Measured by the Bayley Scales of Infant Development? *Behav. Sci.* **2023**, *13*, 542. [CrossRef] [PubMed]

27. Lowe, J.R.; Erickson, S.J.; Schrader, R.; Duncan, A.F. Comparison of the Bayley II Mental Developmental Index and the Bayley III Cognitive Scale: Are We Measuring the Same Thing? *Acta Paediatr.* **2011**, *101*, e55–e58. [CrossRef] [PubMed]
28. Pavlova, P.; Maksimov, D.; Chegodaev, D.; Kiselev, S. A Psychometric Study of the Russian-Language Version of the "Bayley Scales of Infant and Toddler Development–Third Edition": An Assessment of Reliability and Validity. *Front. Psychol.* **2022**, *13*, 961567. [CrossRef] [PubMed]
29. Raghupathy, M.K.; Rao, B.K.; Nayak, S.R.; Spittle, A.J.; Parsekar, S.S. Effect of family-centered care interventions on motor and neurobehavior development of very preterm infants: A protocol for systematic review. *Syst. Rev.* **2021**, *10*, 59. [CrossRef]
30. Morgan, A.S.; Mendonça, M.; Thiele, N.; David, A.L. Management and Outcomes of Extreme Preterm Birth. *BMJ* **2022**, *376*, e055924. [CrossRef]
31. Soleimani, F.; Azari, N.; Ghiasvand, H.; Shahrokhi, A.; Rahmani, N.; Fatollahierad, S. Do NICU Developmental Care Improve Cognitive and Motor Outcomes for Preterm Infants? A Systematic Review and Meta-Analysis. *BMC Pediatr.* **2020**, *20*, 67. [CrossRef]
32. Eichner, J.M.; Johnson, B.H.; Betts, J.M.; Chitkara, M.B.; Jewell, J.A.; Lye, P.S.; Mirkinson, L.J.; Brown, C.; Heiss, K.; Lostocco, L.; et al. Patient- and Family-Centered Care and the Pediatrician's Role. *Pediatrics* **2012**, *129*, 394–404. [CrossRef]
33. Fernandes, A.K.; Wilson, S.; Nalin, A.P.; Philip, A.; Gruber, L.; Kwizera, E.; Sydelko, B.S.; Forbis, S.G.; Lauden, S. Pediatric Family-Centered Rounds and Humanism: A Systematic Review and Qualitative Meta-Analysis. *Hosp. Pediatr.* **2021**, *11*, 636–649. [CrossRef] [PubMed]
34. Del Rosario, C.; Slevin, M.; Molloy, E.J.; Quigley, J.; Nixon, E. How to Use the Bayley Scales of Infant and Toddler Development. *Arch. Dis. Child.-Educ. Pract.* **2021**, *106*, 108–112. [CrossRef] [PubMed]
35. Baxter, S.; Johnson, M.; Chambers, D.; Sutton, A.; Goyder, E.; Booth, A. The Effects of Integrated Care: A Systematic Review of UK and International Evidence. *BMC Health Serv. Res.* **2018**, *18*, 350. [CrossRef] [PubMed]
36. Klein, V.; Zores-Koenig, C.; Dillenseger, L.; Langlet, C.; Escande, B.; Astruc, D.; Le Ray, I.; Kuhn, P. Changes of Infant- and Family-Centered Care Practices Administered to Extremely Preterm Infants During Implementation of the NIDCAP Program. *Front. Pediatr.* **2021**, *9*, 718813. [CrossRef] [PubMed]
37. Dean, S.; Long, M.; Ryan, E.; Tarnoviski, K.; Mondal, A.; Lisanti, A.J. Assessment of an Educational Tool for Pediatric Cardiac Nurses on Individualized Family-Centered Developmental Care. *Crit. Care Nurse* **2021**, *41*, e17–e27. [CrossRef] [PubMed]
38. Kuo, D.Z.; Houtrow, A.J.; Arango, P.; Kuhlthau, K.A.; Simmons, J.M.; Neff, J.M. Family-Centered Care: Current Applications and Future Directions in Pediatric Health Care. *Matern. Child Health J.* **2012**, *16*, 297–305. [CrossRef]
39. Kokorelias, K.M.; Gignac, M.A.M.; Naglie, G.; Cameron, J.I. Towards a Universal Model of Family Centered Care: A Scoping Review. *BMC Health Serv. Res.* **2019**, *19*, 564. [CrossRef]
40. Knighton, A.J.; Bass, E.J. Implementing Family-Centered Rounds in Hospital Pediatric Settings: A Scoping Review. *Hosp. Pediatr.* **2021**, *11*, 679–691. [CrossRef]
41. Ortinau, C.M.; Smyser, C.D.; Arthur, L.; Gordon, E.E.; Heydarian, H.C.; Wolovits, J.; Nedrelow, J.; Marino, B.S.; Levy, V.Y. Optimizing Neurodevelopmental Outcomes in Neonates with Congenital Heart Disease. *Pediatrics* **2022**, *150*, e2022056415L. [CrossRef]
42. Brumbaugh, J.E.; Bell, E.F.; Do, B.T.; Greenberg, R.G.; Stoll, B.J.; DeMauro, S.B.; Harmon, H.M.; Hintz, S.R.; Das, A.; Puopolo, K.M.; et al. Incidence of and Neurodevelopmental Outcomes after Late-Onset Meningitis among Children Born Extremely Preterm. *JAMA Netw. Open* **2022**, *5*, e2245826. [CrossRef]

children

MDPI

Article

Parenting Influences on Frontal Lobe Gray Matter and Preterm Toddlers' Problem-Solving Skills

Josselyn S. Muñoz [1,†], Megan E. Giles [2,†], Kelly A. Vaughn [2], Ying Wang [2], Susan H. Landry [2], Johanna R. Bick [3] and Dana M. DeMaster [2,*]

[1] Department of Cognitive Sciences, Rice University, Houston, TX 77005, USA; josselyn.munoz@bcm.edu
[2] Children's Learning Institute, The University of Texas Health Science Center at Houston, Houston, TX 77030, USA; megan.e.giles@uth.tmc.edu (M.E.G.); kelly.a.vaughn@uth.tmc.edu (K.A.V.); ying.wang@uth.tmc.edu (Y.W.); susan.landry@uth.tmc.edu (S.H.L.)
[3] Psychology Department, University of Houston, Houston, TX 77204, USA; jrbick@uh.edu
* Correspondence: dana.m.demaster@uth.tmc.edu
† These authors contributed equally to this work.

Abstract: Children born preterm often face challenges with self-regulation during toddlerhood. This study examined the relationship between prematurity, supportive parent behaviors, frontal lobe gray matter volume (GMV), and emotion regulation (ER) among toddlers during a parent-assisted, increasingly complex problem-solving task, validated for this age range. Data were collected from preterm toddlers (n = 57) ages 15–30 months corrected for prematurity and their primary caregivers. MRI data were collected during toddlers' natural sleep. The sample contained three gestational groups: 22–27 weeks (extremely preterm; EPT), 28–33 weeks (very preterm; VPT), and 34–36 weeks (late preterm; LPT). Older toddlers became more compliant as the Tool Task increased in difficulty, but this pattern varied by gestational group. Engagement was highest for LPT toddlers, for older toddlers, and for the easiest task condition. Parents did not differentiate their support depending on task difficulty or their child's age or gestational group. Older children had greater frontal lobe GMV, and for EPT toddlers only, more parent support was related to larger right frontal lobe GMV. We found that parent support had the greatest impact on high birth risk (≤27 gestational weeks) toddler brain development, thus early parent interventions may normalize preterm child neurodevelopment and have lasting impacts.

Keywords: prematurity; neurodevelopment; neuroimaging; parenting; emotion regulation; cognition; frontal lobe; gray matter volume

1. Introduction

Medical advances have improved the survival rate and physical needs of very preterm infants (VPT; less than 33 gestational weeks), but children born preterm continue to have elevated risk for neurodevelopmental difficulties (e.g., executive function, emotion regulation, language, etc.) [1–4]. These observed neurodevelopmental difficulties may result from brain injury at birth and/or disruption in utero brain development [5–9]. Early experiences, including duration and medical care in the neonatal intensive care unit (NICU) and parenting behaviors may also influence neurodevelopmental outcomes following preterm birth [10–12].

Parents play an important role in neurodevelopmental outcomes for children born preterm. Providing warm and contingent caregiving, which responds to the child's attentional cues and meets their needs, has been associated with improved social–emotional and cognitive functioning in preterm-born children [13,14]. In addition, there is evidence that parental responsiveness directly influences the development of prefrontal gray matter with strong implications for improving self-regulation in children born VPT. For example, higher levels of parental sensitivity in early childhood are associated with larger total brain volume, as well as gray matter volume at 8 years [15]. Similarly, parental responsiveness may lead to better amygdala and prefrontal gray matter neurodevelopment, with the ultimate effect of reducing the risk of emotion regulation (ER) disruption and psychopathology among children. Yet, less is known regarding the effects of parental responsiveness on frontal limbic development and regulatory skills in children born preterm [16]. Taken together, the studies emphasize the importance of warm and responsive caregiving in optimizing neurodevelopmental outcomes for children, particularly those born preterm.

Early childhood is a crucial period marked by significant cognitive development, which serves as a foundational element for more nuanced cognitive functions later in life [17]. Self-regulation, or the ability to regulate one's behavior in relation to what is environmentally appropriate, is contingent on executive functioning (EF) and emotion regulation (ER) [18]. Skills that prove vital for self-regulation are shaped during the first two years of life, and the emergence of these skills is intimately linked to development of prefrontal circuits [19,20]. Specifically, the prefrontal–limbic system, including frontostriatal connections, rapidly develops in the first three postnatal years. There is growing evidence that early self-regulatory dysfunction puts preterm children at increased risk for school failure and special education needs, as shown by teacher reports of behavioral and general academic delays [21–23].

Neuroimaging studies consistently link premature birth, particularly occurring before 33 weeks of gestation, with significant atypical white and gray matter microstructure [24]. Even at their term-corrected age, preterm infants exhibit reduced regional brain volumes. The prefrontal cortices that facilitate EF and ER skills encompass various frontal brain regions such as the anterior cingulate, as well as the medial, dorsal, and ventral prefrontal cortex [25]. Consistent with the idea that neural circuitry is most responsive to experience during rapid development, the protracted developmental course of the prefrontal cortex causes these networks to be heavily influenced by experience, and early in life, experiences will primarily stem from caregiver interaction [26–33]. Therefore, EF and ER typically develop in the context of relationships with caregivers and are facilitated by establishing a sense of safety and security, forming secure attachments, and coregulating emotions [34–37].

Within the context of prematurity, NICU stay length and clinical practices are an important environmental factor that shape developmental outcomes. Prolonged NICU stays have been associated with lower scores on the Bayley mental and motor scales during toddlerhood [11]. Interestingly, in this study, gestational age was not associated with the Bayley scales, suggesting that the severity of postnatal illnesses and NICU hospitalization may account for negative neurodevelopmental effects in already high-risk preterm infants. Increasingly, modifiable clinical care factors that may be at play include nutrition and sensory exposure, which are highlighted as targets for improved developmental outcome [12,38]. Moreover, limited parent–infant bonding during extended NICU stays may interfere with formation of secure attachment relationship.

In order to measure and operationalize toddler ER, a task must include challenging elements that require the child to regulate their emotions often in the context of problem solving. The Tool Task was designed to measure aspects of early childhood problem-solving, decision-making, spatial awareness, and emotion regulation, as the child works on increasingly difficult tasks to remove toys from apparatuses with parent support [39]. This task was originally used to evaluate two-year-olds' capacity to engage in ER, sustained attention, and problem-solving behaviors. Importantly, the Tool Task captures the toddler behavior within the context of increasingly complex challenges and measures the child's ability to draw upon personal and environmental resources, such as their caregiver. This task also evaluates parenting behaviors as the extent to which caregivers provide supportive presence and quality of assistance as they work to help the child solve the task on their own.

Consistent with this idea, children classified as having a secure attachment to their primary caregivers showed more enthusiasm, positive affect, persistence, cooperation, flexibility, resourcefulness, and engagement than insecurely attached children. Moreover, higher supportive caregiver behaviors during the task predicted lower negative child behaviors, including frustration, negative affect, and noncompliance behaviors [39]. During Tool Task levels, parental support and responsive behaviors are essential components of parent–child interactions, assessed by the scales of Supportive Presence and Quality of Assistance. These behaviors underscore a caregiver's ability to provide support and assistance to a child during problem-solving situations, contributing significantly to the child's positive and enjoyable learning experiences.

Supportive presence involves the parent's attentiveness to the child and task, coupled with emotional responsiveness to the child's signals. This creates a secure base for exploration, which is achieved by the parent staying calm, setting a positive mood, and being physically present. For example, the parent approaches the tool with obvious interest and enthusiasm. The parent makes certain that the child realizes there is a problem to be solved and indicates to the child that working on the problem can be rewarding. The parent may also indicate to the child that they are available to work cooperatively with him/her if it becomes necessary but encourages initial autonomous work to help the child achieve a sense of solving the problem her/himself. These supportive behaviors not only motivate but also reassure the child, leading to a high score on the Supportive Presence scale.

The current study examined the consequences of prematurity on frontal lobe gray matter volume (GMV) and emotion regulation (ER) among toddlers engaged in the Tool Task. This study tested associations between parent and child behaviors, with a special emphasis on toddler emotion regulation and parental support facilitated through coregulation, and toddler frontal lobe neurodevelopment for toddlers with varying levels of birth risk (i.e., extremely preterm, EPT; very preterm, VPT; and late preterm, LPT). The following hypotheses were tested: (1) We hypothesized that toddler ER during the Tool Task would vary based on interactive influences of birth risk, task difficulty, and toddler age. Specifically, we expected that there would be differences in ER between EPT, VPT, and LPT toddlers. (2) In terms of frontal lobe GMV, we anticipated that LPT toddlers would have the greatest frontal lobe GMV and EPT toddlers would have the least frontal lobe GMV. (3) Finally, we hypothesized that parent support would be most beneficial for EPT toddlers, both in terms of child behavior (e.g., more supportive parent behaviors associated with more toddler compliance and engagement) and in terms of frontal lobe GMV (e.g., more supportive parent behaviors associated with greater frontal lobe GMV).

2. Materials and Methods

This study included toddlers born preterm between 15–30 corrected gestational months and their primary caregivers. Sample demographics (n = 57) are presented in Table 1. The research team recruited the participants from two large pediatric clinics affiliated with the University of Texas Health Science Center located at the Texas Medical Center in Houston, TX, USA. Participants included in this sample had completed the initial testing: MRI and Tool Task. MRI data were successfully collected from 35 participants. This study is part of a larger longitudinal study that utilizes scalable parenting interventions to test if parental responsiveness is a modifiable psychological factor that improves neurodevelopmental outcomes and brain connectivity in toddlers born preterm. Tool Task data were collected in a laboratory setting at the Children's Learning Institute in Houston, TX, as part of baseline assessment, and was administered along with other parent reports and behavioral measures for the larger study. Behavioral assessments were video recorded and coded (see Supplementary Materials for coding framework). MRI data were acquired, concurrently with behavioral data, at Baylor College of Medicine Core for Advanced Magnetic Resonance Imaging in Houston, TX. The study participants received a gift card for completing this behavioral testing session. Prior to any testing, informed consent was obtained from all parents involved in this study; children enrolled in this study were too young to provide assent for participation.

Table 1. Descriptive characteristics of participants (n = 57).

Sample Characteristics	n (%)
Child Sex	
Male	30 (52.63)
Female	27 (47.37)
Child Race	
Black or African American	20 (35.09)
White	21 (36.84)
Asian	2 (3.51)
American Indian or Alaska Native	1 (1.75)
Native Hawaiian or Other Pacific Islander	1 (1.75)
Declined to respond	12
Child Ethnicity	
Yes, Hispanic or Latino	30 (52.63)
No, not Hispanic or Latino	24 (42.10)
Declined to respond	3
Gestation Classification	
Extreme Preterm (22–27)	28 (44.92)
Very Preterm (28–33)	15 (26.32)
Late Preterm (34–36)	14 (24.56)
Caregiver Relationship to Child	
Mother	52 (91.2)
Father	4 (7)
Other	1 (1.8)
Caregiver Education: Highest Grade Completed	
Primary school, Finished 5th grade	2 (3.5)
Middle School	4 (7)
Some High School	8 (14)
High School diploma or GED	7 (12.3)
Vocational or technical training	2 (3.5)
Some College	11 (19.3)
Bachelor's degree (BA/BS)	15 (26.3)
Master's degree MA, MS, JD	4 (7)
Other	3 (5.3)
Declined to respond	1 (1.8)
	Means (SD)
Adjusted Gestational Age in months	19.24 (4.904)
Gestational Age at Birth (weeks)	28.60 (4.39)
Primary Caregiver Age	32.74 (7.22)

The study procedure was approved by the Committee for the Protection of Human Subjects at the University of Texas Health Science Center at Houston. The Tool Task was administered according to standard guidelines [39], optimized for our study design. Each child was seated in a booster seat next to their parent at a table. The three levels of the

Tool Task increased in difficulty, increasing the need for emotion regulation and parent assistance while problem-solving (Figure 1a–d). During a 1 to 1.5-h baseline testing session, the Tool Task was the first task administered. The Tool Task had three levels that took between one to four minutes to complete and that increased in difficulty. The first level, "vault toy," asked the child to turn a wheel until the vault unlocked to release the prize (a book) that was inside (Figure 1a). The second level was the "short tube" task, in which the child inserted a stick inside a clear tube to retrieve the toy stuck in the middle (Figure 1b). The third level, the "long tube" task, was similar to the second level (Figure 1c). However, for the third level, the parent and toddler needed to realize that they were not able to release the toy stuck in the middle of the clear tube by using one stick, instead they had to put together both halves of the sticks so that it was long enough to push the toy through the tube. The parent was present for all problem-solving tasks and instructed to let the child try to solve the problem independently, but they were able to provide as much help as they thought their child needed (Figure 1d). These tasks, especially the third level, tended to be stressful, thus requiring child emotion regulation and increased coregulation from parent to child.

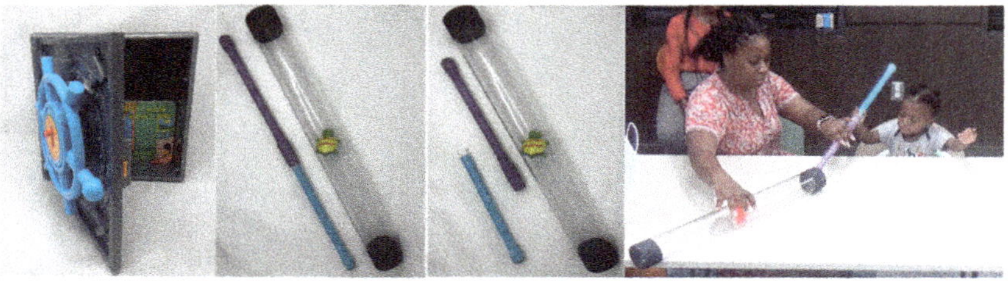

(a) (b) (c) (d)

Figure 1. Tool Task apparatus levels with parent–child interaction. (**a**) Vault toy apparatus corresponding to difficulty Level 1. (**b**) Short tube apparatus corresponding to difficulty level 2. (**c**) Long tube apparatus corresponding to difficulty level 3. (**d**) Mother supporting child well in level 2 of the Tool Task. Notice the parent's hand-over-hand assistance and child's active engagement in the task.

Behavioral coding measures and framework. For each level, three coders analyzed six variables for child behaviors and two variables for caregiver behaviors (interrater reliability, $\alpha = 0.95$). Each of the videos had 24 total ratings across the child and caregiver variables (8 variables per 3 levels). Coders began analyzing behaviors when the examiner put the toy and apparatus on the table and said, "Can you get the toy out of the box or tube?" Coders stopped coding approximately ten seconds after the child retrieved the prize. The only coding exclusion was when the parent was talking to the examiner or other adults in the room. Behavioral coding materials are included in Supplementary Materials.

Child behavioral measures. Child *noncompliance* was measured on a 1 to 6 scale evaluating the extent to which the child attended to the caregiver and complied with caregiver requests. A high score would mean more noncompliance as shown by the child refusing all caregiver offers of support and never following caregiver directions. A low score, in contrast, means that the child attended to most of the parent's requests and followed the instructions. Child *engagement* was measured on a scale of 1–7 and was defined as the degree to which the child is interested, engaged in, and enthusiastic about the task. A score of 1 reflects the child's active effort to avoid the task, whereas a score of 7 reflects very high levels of engagement and thorough involvement in the task, and the middle of the scale reflects moderate levels of engagement. Other child behaviors did not have enough variability to examine (see Table 2).

Table 2. Gestational group differences in behavioral measures of the Tool Task using ANCOVA, with age as a covariate.

Measure	Extremely Preterm	Very Preterm	Late Preterm	F(df)	p
	Means (SE)	Means (SE)	Means (SE)		
Child Behavioral Measures					
Child Noncompliance					
Level 1	2.824 (0.277)	2.946 (0.360)	2.523 (0.373)	0.350 (2,46)	0.707
Level 2	3.210 (0.294)	3.795 (0.382)	3.080 (0.395)	1.005 (2,46)	0.374
Level 3	4.127 (0.281)	3.682 (0.365)	3.734 (0.377)	0.608 (2,46)	0.549
Child Anger +					
Level 1	1.044 (0.193)	1.421 (0.251)	1.392 (0.260)	0.954 (2,46)	0.393
Level 2	1.083 (0.198)	1.470 (0.257)	1.886 (0.266)	3.012 (2,46)	0.059
Level 3	1.564 (0.292)	1.373 (0.380)	2.140 (0.393)	1.065 (2,46)	0.353
Child Coping +					
Level 1	2.869 (0.157)	3.220 (0.204)	3.380 (0.211)	2.158 (2,46)	0.127
Level 2	2.781 (0.178)	3.015 (0.231)	3.140 (0.239)	0.809 (2,46)	0.452
Level 3	2.607 (0.172)	2.946 (0.223)	2.907 (0.231)	0.945 (2,46)	0.396
Child Engagement					
Level 1	3.921 (0.259)	3.776 (0.337)	5.151 (0.349)	5.018 (2,46)	0.011 *
Level 2	4.010 (0.299)	3.394 (0.388)	4.865 (0.401)	3.418 (2,46)	0.041 *
Level 3	3.191 (0.299)	3.539 (0.388)	4.620 (0.401)	4.145 (2,46)	0.022 *
Child Persistence +					
Level 1	3.176 (0.241)	3.193 (0.313)	4.019 (0.324)	2.455 (2,46)	0.097
Level 2	3.225 (0.266)	2.634 (0.346)	3.612 (0.357)	1.941 (2,46)	0.155
Level 3	2.660 (0.249)	2.846 (0.323)	3.383 (0.335)	1.520 (2,46)	0.229
Parent Assistance Sum					
Level 1	10.500 (0.615)	9.911 (0.799)	11.672 (0.827)	1.195 (2,46)	0.312
Level 2	11.017 (0.527)	9.888 (0.685)	11.705 (0.708)	1.720 (2,46)	0.190
Level 3	10.271 (0.522)	10.109 (0.678)	12.173 (0.702)	2.884 (2,46)	0.066
Across Levels				3.84 (2,46)	0.029 *

+ not hypothesized or included in analyses; * $p < 0.05$.

Caregiver behavioral measures. Coders observed the supportive presence and quality of assistance from the caregiver. Using a 1 to 7 scale, coders rated the emotional support with which the parent helped the child have a positive learning experience. Higher ratings meant that the parent met most criteria and subcriteria (providing secure base, attentiveness to child, helping their child focus, reinforcing, staying calm, anticipating frustration, setting a learning and enjoyable mood, etc.). The quality of assistance measure also used a 1 to 7 scale to evaluate the sensitivity with which the caregiver maximized the child's learning opportunities. If the caregiver received the highest score, then they were excellent at giving assistance. To show the combination of warmth and contingent responsiveness, we summed the two parent variables in the analysis for an overview of their level of assistance provided (i.e., Parent Assistance + Parent Supportive Presence = Parent Assistance Sum).

Toddler MRI Scans. MRI data were collected within seven days on average after the behavioral data (36% on the same day) during the toddlers' natural sleep. T1 and T2 weighted images were collected using a 64-channel head coil on a Siemens 3T scanner. The parents were instructed to perform their usual bedtime routine with the child and to alert the research staff once the child had been asleep for fifteen minutes. Then, researchers transferred the child from the bed into the scanner. Hearing protection included earplugs, pediatric earmuffs, and a thick piece of foam curved around the interior of the bore to act similar to an acoustic hood [40]. A member of the research team was inside the scanner, monitoring the child for movement and distress. If the child awoke, the scan was stopped immediately.

The T1 and T2 scans were processed using Infant Brain Extraction and Analysis Toolbox (iBEAT V2.0 Cloud) for initial processing and brain segmentation [41–45]. The neuroimaging processing steps included the following: heterogeneity correction, skull stripping, and tissue segmentation. FSL was then used for gray matter volume computation to calculate total gray matter volume and gray matter volume within each parcellation of the UNC-BCP 4D Infant Brain Volumetric Atlas (Figure 2) [46]. All frontal regions included in analyses are presented in Table 3. There was no significant difference between the right and left frontal gray matter volumes ($t(34) = 1.94$, $p = 0.06$).

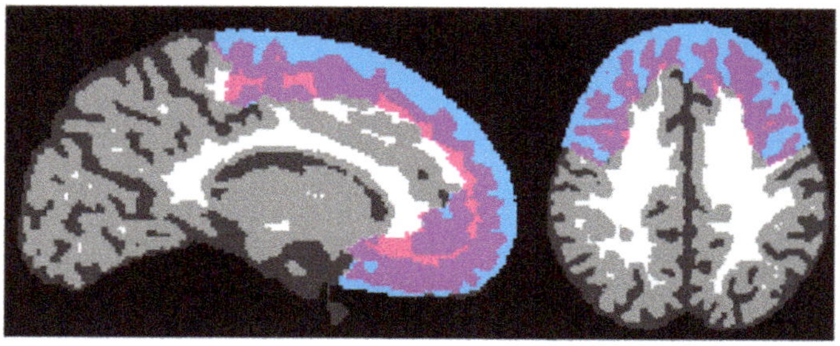

Figure 2. iBEAT brain segmentation example. The blue represents cerebrospinal fluid, the purple is gray matter, and the pink is white matter.

Table 3. Gestational group differences in frontal gray matter using ANCOVA, with age and total gray matter volume as covariates.

Measure	Extremely Preterm	Very Preterm	Late Preterm	*F(df)*	*p*
	Means (SE)	**Means (SE)**	**Means (SE)**		
Left Frontal Gray Matter Regional Volumes					
Sum of frontal regions	58,678 (1056)	58,346 (1427)	60,719 (1354)	0.911 (2,30)	0.413
Middle frontal gyrus	10,261 (367)	10,743 (497)	10,803 (471)	0.533 (2,30)	0.592
Precentral gyrus	7228 (236)	7197 (319)	7691 (303)	0.867 (2,30)	0.430
Supplementary motor area	4172 (169)	4137 (229)	4342 (217)	0.255 (2,30)	0.776
Medial orbitofrontal cortex	1506 (107)	1421 (144)	1424 (137)	0.165 (2,30)	0.849
Inf. orbitofrontal cortex	4181 (223)	4306 (301)	5003 (286)	2.684 (2,30)	0.085
Middle orbitofrontal cortex	1915 (123)	1580 (166)	2161 (158)	3.147 (2,30)	0.057
Medial sup. frontal gyrus	5093 (279)	4920 (377)	4914 (358)	0.107 (2,30)	0.898
Dorsal sup. frontal gyrus	5455 (230)	5581 (311)	5439 (296)	0.067 (2,30)	0.935
Rolandic operculum	3649 (71)	3513 (96)	3738 (91)	1.436 (2,30)	0.254
Triangular inf. frontal gyrus	6521 (171)	6226 (231)	6788 (219)	1.522 (2,30)	0.235
Opercular inf. frontal gyrus	2450 (69)	2452 (93)	2594 (88)	0.930 (2,30)	0.405
Rectus gyrus	1792 (198)	2029 (268)	1365 (254)	1.662 (2,30)	0.207
Anterior cingulate cortex	4455 (147)	4243 (199)	4457 (189)	0.422 (2,30)	0.660

Table 3. *Cont.*

Measure	Extremely Preterm	Very Preterm	Late Preterm	*F(df)*	*p*
	Means (SE)	Means (SE)	Means (SE)		
Right Frontal Gray Matter Regional Volumes					
Sum of frontal regions	59,944 (1460)	59,620 (1973)	63,532 (1973)	1.386 (2,30)	0.266
Middle frontal gyrus	10,241 (486)	10,323 (657)	10,950 (623)	0.427 (2,30)	0.656
Precentral gyrus	7219 (307)	7291 (416)	7849 (394)	0.844 (2,30)	0.440
Supplementary motor area	4356 (175)	4748 (236)	4762 (224)	1.411 (2,30)	0.260
Medial orbitofrontal cortex	2159 (113)	2075 (152)	2259 (144)	0.379 (2,30)	0.688
Inf. orbitofrontal cortex	4638 (198)	4341 (267)	5202 (254)	2.824 (2,30)	0.075
Middle orbitofrontal cortex	2348 (163)	1958 (221)	2743 (209)	3.254 (2,30)	0.053
Medial sup. frontal gyrus	3252 (242)	3423 (327)	3253 (310)	0.100 (2,30)	0.905
Dorsal sup. frontal gyrus	6383 (301)	6266 (407)	6458 (386)	0.058 (2,30)	0.944
Rolandic operculum	4618 (75)	4386 (101)	4624 (96)	1.967 (2,30)	0.157
Triangular inf. frontal gyrus	4798 (116)	4538 (157)	5238 (149)	5.316 (2,30)	0.011 *
Opercular inf. frontal gyrus	3678 (123)	3768 (166)	3885 (158)	0.541 (2,30)	0.588
Rectus gyrus	1708 (191)	1864 (258)	1488 (245)	0.557 (2,30)	0.579
Anterior cingulate cortex	4546 (144)	4642 (195)	4822 (185)	0.686 (2,30)	0.511

* $p < 0.05$.

Statistical Analysis. We conducted linear mixed effects models with task difficulty (levels 1, 2, and 3) as a within-subjects variable and gestational group (EPT, VPT, and LPT) and age (adjusted for prematurity) as between-subjects variables. We used these models to predict toddler and parent behavior during the Tool Task. To examine brain structure differences across gestational groups, we conducted linear mixed effects models with hemisphere (right/left) as a within-subjects variable and gestational group (EPT, VPT, and LPT) and age (adjusted for prematurity) as between-subjects variables, controlling for total GMV. We also explored the relationships between parent behaviors during the Tool Task, child behaviors during the Tool Task, and bilateral frontal lobe GMV. A power sensitivity analysis was performed using G*Power version 3.1 [47]. With a sample size (N) of 57 and three gestational groups, the study demonstrates a relative effect size ranging from 0.423 to 0.546, ensuring a statistical power (1-β err prob) of 0.80 and 0.95 [48].

3. Results

Descriptive statistics for all Tool Task outcome variables by gestational group are presented in Table 2, with age included as a covariate. Birth risk was unrelated to parent assistance and toddler noncompliance, anger, coping, and persistence during the Tool Task. There was a significant difference in toddler engagement across the gestational groups: in all three levels of the Tool Task, LPT toddlers were more engaged than VPT or EPT toddlers.

3.1. Toddler Noncompliance

There was a significant three-way interaction between gestational group, task difficulty, and adjusted age ($F(4,88) = 3.23$, $p = 0.02$). The pattern generally reflects increased compliance for older toddlers as the task increased in difficulty, but this relationship differed by gestational group (see Figure 3). For LPT toddlers, who had the lowest birth risk, older toddlers were more compliant than younger toddlers at level 3 of the Tool Task only; there was no relationship between compliance and age for levels 1 and 2. For VPT toddlers, who had moderate birth risk, older toddlers were more compliant than younger toddlers at levels 2 and 3 of the Tool Task; there was no relationship between compliance and age for level 1. For EPT toddlers, who had the highest birth risk, older toddlers were more compliant than younger toddlers at level 1 of the Tool Task only; there was no relationship between compliance and age for levels 2 and 3.

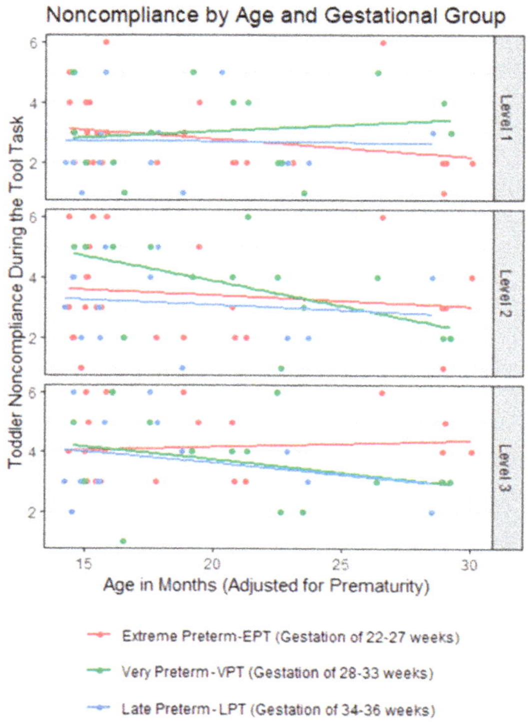

Figure 3. Toddler noncompliance by levels (1–3) of the Tool Task and three gestational groups.

3.2. Toddler Engagement

The three-way interaction between gestational group, task difficulty, and adjusted age was not significant for toddler engagement during the Tool Task ($F(4,88) = 2.035$, $p = 0.10$). There was a significant main effect of task difficulty ($F(2,88) = 3.84$, $p = 0.03$) and a significant main effect of adjusted age ($F(1,44) = 5.04$, $p = 0.03$). Engagement decreased with task difficulty and increased with age.

3.3. Parent Support

Parents did not differentiate their support during the Tool Task depending on their child's age ($F(1,46) = 2.43$, $p = 0.13$), their child's gestational group ($F(2,46) = 1.93$, $p = 0.16$), or task difficulty ($F(2,45) = 1.52$, $p = 0.22$).

3.4. Parent Support and Toddler Noncompliance

Because parent support did not differ by task difficulty, we created a sum score to represent overall parent support across all three levels of the task (see Table 2). In a model predicting toddler noncompliance from parent support, gestational group, and age, toddler noncompliance was not related to overall parent support ($F(1,45) = 2.33$, $p = 0.13$).

3.5. Parent Support and Toddler Engagement

In a model predicting toddler engagement from parent support, gestational group, and age, there was significant interaction between parent support and gestational group ($F(2,43) = 5.23$, $p = 0.01$). To better understand this interaction, exploratory univariate analyses were conducted for each gestational group, testing main effects of parent support on child engagement within each level, such that effect of parenting support at each task level was tested relative to child behavior at the same task level. Univariate results indicated that EPT toddlers who received more parent support were more engaged ($F(1,22) = 6.75$, $p = 0.02$) at level 2; whereas, for LPT toddlers parental support predicted child engagement at level 3 ($F(1,10) = 8.39$, $p = 0.02$). Parent support did not predict child engagement for VPT toddlers. Of note, a summed score of parent support was evaluated in the primary analysis, which was appropriate for testing differences in child behavior across levels. However, to evaluate child behavior within each task level, a level-specific score for parent support was deemed more suitable.

3.6. Frontal Lobe GMV

Frontal lobe GMV was unrelated to the gestational group ($F(2,28) = 0.60$, $p = 0.62$). Across gestational groups, older children had greater frontal lobe GMV than younger children ($F(1,28) = 12.24$, $p = 0.002$).

3.7. Frontal Lobe GMV and Parent Support

At levels 2 and 3, there was a significant interaction between gestational group and parent support in predicting right frontal lobe GMV (level 2: $F(3,22) = 4.27$, $p = 0.01$; level 3: $F(3,21) = 6.17$, $p = 0.004$). The interaction indicated that parent support was related to right frontal lobe GMV only for EPT toddlers; EPT toddlers with parents who were more supportive during the Tool Task had greater right frontal lobe GMV than EPT toddlers with parents who were less supportive during the Tool Task (see Figure 4). Parent support was unrelated to frontal lobe GMV for VPT and LPT toddlers. There were no significant interactions between gestational group and parent support for the left frontal lobe GMV.

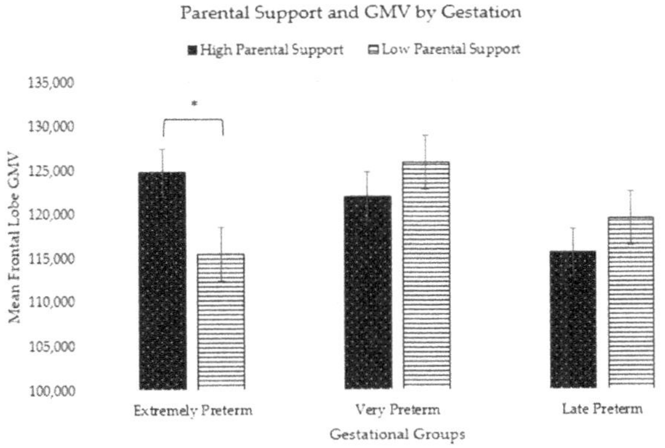

Figure 4. Graph of parental support and GMV by gestation shows the significant effect of high parental support on EPT child frontal GMV. * $p < 0.05$.

3.8. NICU Stay Length

The current study analyzed the duration of NICU stay in days and its potential impact on GMV and ER. Results showed a non-significant effect of NICU stay duration on total GMV or frontal GMV ($Fs(1,34) \leq 0.35$, $ps \geq 0.56$). The effect of NICU stay duration on toddler ER throughout the three levels of the Tool Task was also nonsignificant ($Fs(1,53) \leq 3.45$, $ps \geq 0.07$).

4. Discussion

Previous research indicates that utilizing brain plasticity during the critical period of toddlerhood can serve as a mechanism to promote healthy developmental outcomes for preterm (PT) children [34]. Responsive interactions with caregivers have the potential to enhance neurodevelopmental outcomes, including cognition, language, and brain microstructure, for children at risk of cognitive, psychiatric, and behavioral disorders, particularly those born extremely premature [33]. Both healthy toddlers and those born preterm are at a pivotal stage in neurodevelopment, wherein environmental stimuli, especially parenting, must be adaptively responsive to address each child's evolving needs. This adaptability is crucial for fostering positive neurodevelopmental outcomes. The reciprocal interaction between parents and toddlers during play, as well as routine activities such as grocery shopping and dressing, provides the necessary stimulation for the healthy development of brain regions associated with emerging language, cognitive skills, and emotion regulation capacities. Taking a step further, actively supporting brain development, particularly in the frontal lobes, through responsive parenting could be a key factor in improving neurodevelopmental outcomes among extremely preterm individuals, who frequently encounter challenges related to frontal lobe processes such as executive function (EF) and emotion regulation (ER).

This study makes a significant contribution to the existing literature by illustrating the positive impact of responsive parenting on brain development, leading to increased gray matter volume (GMV) in the frontal lobe of extremely preterm toddlers. Supporting our hypothesis, older toddlers were more compliant as the Tool Task became harder. One possibility is that, across gestational groups, older toddlers are better able work as a team with their caregivers to solve difficult problems—that is to say, older toddlers are better able inhibit their own agenda to make use of caregiver supports and suggestions. Regarding gestational effects, LPT toddlers are more compliant only in the third level, but at moderate level difficulty older VPT toddlers were more compliant at levels 2 and 3. EPT toddlers showed a similar pattern, but only at level 1, the easiest level of the task. Regardless of age, EPT toddlers were moderately noncompliant throughout levels 2 and 3. This pattern reflects the perception of difficulty for each gestational group, as EPT toddlers find it difficult at level 1, VPT toddlers find it difficult at level 2, and LPT toddlers find it difficult at level 3. This effect may be due to the lower birth risk allowing for typical developmental patterns to become evident at this age.

Supporting our hypothesis, child engagement decreased as the task became more challenging, but increased with child age. It is likely that the frustration inherent to increased task difficulty leading led to lower engagement, although older children were better able to regulate negative emotions and allocate attention to achieving the goal, leading to higher engagement across difficulty levels. Like the age-related effects, LPT toddlers exhibited the highest levels of engagement across all task levels, possibly owing to their ability to employ emotion regulation, enabling them to focus on the task goals. Exploratory analysis suggests that parent support is an individual difference; thus, the absence of differences in parent support may be attributed to consistent personality traits rather than the state of assisting the child during problem-solving.

Whereas parent support was not related to toddler noncompliance, it did impact toddler engagement. LPT and EPT toddlers with supportive parents demonstrated higher engagement in the task. Importantly, the effects of parent support on child engagement were noticeable at level 3 for LPT toddlers and level 2 for EPT toddlers, underscoring the need for parental support to be adaptively tailored to meet the changing needs of toddlers. The observed patterns of child engagement and parent support in challenging tasks align with the concept of scaffolding in Vygotsky's sociocultural theory. Within the caregiving context, Vygotsky's scaffolding principal centers on providing support and guidance to a learner, adjusting the level of assistance as needed. EPT and LPT toddlers, possibly due to their specific developmental readiness, may benefit from more effective parental scaffolding at level 2 and level 3, respectively, facilitating their engagement and success at an appropriate point in this challenging task [49,50].

Frontal lobe GMV only differed by age, where older children had greater GMV than younger children due to increased neurodevelopment as they age. The differences by age are similar across the three groups as expected. In line with our hypothesis that parent support benefits high birth risk toddlers the most, there was an interaction between gestational group and parent support, such that the high birth risk group (EPT) showed greater right frontal lobe GMV with greater parent support. It is unclear why parenting effects were right lateralized, one possibility is that right frontal lobe may be more involved in ER and thus more malleable to environment specific stimulation, such as parenting behavior [51]; whereas left frontal lobe may be more sensitive to other environmental factors, such as rich language exposure. Although the constrained sample size of this study warrants caution, it is essential to consider the finding that parental behavior impacted the frontal lobe GMV in the gestational group at the highest neurodevelopmental risk (i.e., EPT). This finding aligns with the differential susceptibility theoretical framework [52], which suggests that individuals more susceptible to adversity may also be more responsive to positive influences, such as supportive parenting. Within the context of prematurity, according to this framework, those at the highest neurodevelopmental risk may benefit the most from supportive parenting practices. Consistent with our hypothesis, EPT toddlers who received substantial parental support during the task exhibited significantly greater gray matter volume in the frontal lobe. This EPT group experienced the most atypical developmental journey and longest postnatal period, distinguishing them from the later gestational groups. In this cohort with the highest birth risk, parental support appears to play a crucial role in mitigating GMV deficiencies among preterm children, potentially contributing to improved cognitive and socioemotional development and lowering the risk of psychiatric disorders. Subsequent research, including a larger sample and longitudinal design, should delve into the effects of parental intervention on preterm toddler GMV, emotion regulation, and the intricate interplay with parental support.

Present findings highlighting the significant influence of parent support on the brain development of toddlers at the highest birth risk are compelling but should be considered within the context of the following limitations. First, to achieve these study aims, multiple hypotheses were tested on a relatively small sample size, increasing the risk for false positives. Toddlers born with low gestational ages (EPT and VPT) constitute a specialized population, which increases the potential impact of research findings; yet researchers working *with* pediatric patient populations and their families are aware of health-related (e.g., ongoing outpatient therapies, respiratory illness) barriers for recruitment and enrollment, ultimately limiting sample size. For this reason, the modest sample size in this study necessitates cautious interpretation of results. Future studies with larger samples are recommended to enhance generalizability and robustness of findings. Furthermore, the cross-sectional nature of this study does not capture developmental change over time. Instead, our study design allows for the inference of age-related changes in both brain and behavior, alongside current environmental experience. Future longitudinal studies are essential to provide a more comprehensive understanding of the dynamic developmental and even infer differential trajectories of brain–behavior outcomes in preterm toddlers.

The inclusion of MRI data in this research provides valuable insights into the intricate relationship between brain development and behavioral outcomes in toddlers born preterm. Although the acquisition of MRI data from sleeping toddlers represents an innovative approach, it is important to note that a limitation was that frontal lobe volumetric analyses were restricted to toddlers who remained asleep during MRI data acquisition. This limitation might introduce bias, as our sample could be skewed toward toddlers who experience less disruption during natural sleep. An anecdotal note of interest—investigators in this study collect several variables on child sleep habits. Surprisingly, sensitivity to sound during sleep and regular bedtime are not sufficient predictors of success; whereas, multiple MRI data collection attempts and same day behavioral and MRI testing support MRI data acquisition. One final limitation, the study did not assess motor skill ability or milestones, and it is plausible that EPT and VPT toddlers faced additional challenges in this domain compared to LPT toddlers. While the Tool Task's coding framework allows for scaling of coded behaviors based on child capacity, future investigations should consider incorporating fine motor skill assessments to provide a more comprehensive understanding of the interplay between parenting behaviors, emotion regulation, and motor development challenges in preterm infants and toddlers.

5. Conclusions

Based on our results that parent support has the greatest impact on the highest birth risk (under 28 weeks gestation) toddler brain development, parent interventions may be warranted to normalize their child's brain development from the start and create a lasting positive impact. Future work research should target increasing positive parenting behavior to improve brain development, ER, and other cognitive skills in toddlers born preterm. Continuing to investigate the effects of parenting interventions on preterm toddlers could establish the way for this population to have better ER/EF mechanisms and reach their full developmental potential.

Supplementary Materials: The following supporting information can be downloaded at: https://www.mdpi.com/article/10.3390/children11020206/s1.

Author Contributions: Conceptualization, D.M.D., M.E.G., J.S.M., J.R.B., Y.W. and S.H.L.; methodology, D.M.D., J.R.B. and S.H.L.; formal analysis, D.M.D.; resources, D.M.D., J.R.B. and S.H.L.; data curation, M.E.G.; writing—original draft preparation, M.E.G. and J.S.M.; writing—review and editing, K.A.V., D.M.D. and Y.W.; coding framework adaption and coding, M.E.G. and Y.W.; visualization, M.E.G. and K.A.V.; supervision, D.M.D. and S.H.L.; funding acquisition, D.M.D., J.R.B., K.A.V. and S.H.L. All authors have read and agreed to the published version of the manuscript.

Funding: This research was funded by the Eunice Kennedy Shriver National Institute of Child Health and Human Development, grant number R01HD100560. The APC was funded by this NIH award.

Institutional Review Board Statement: The study was conducted in accordance with the Declaration of Helsinki, and approved by the Institutional Review Board (or Ethics Committee) of The University of Texas Health Science Center at Houston (IRB number: HSC-MS-17-0190, IRB approval date: 29 September 2023).

Informed Consent Statement: Informed consent was obtained from all subjects involved in the study. Specifically, written informed consent had been obtained from the patients' primary caregiver prior to publishing of this paper. Media consent was obtained from family modeling Tool Task in Figure 1.

Data Availability Statement: Data are contained within the article and Supplementary Materials.

Acknowledgments: A special thank you to Li Wang for support implementing MRI data parcellations in iBEAT V2.0: Infant Brain Extraction and Analysis Toolbox. Additional thank you to Texas Advanced Computing Center (https://tacc.utexas.edu (accessed on 30 January 2024)) for technical assistance with utilizing IBEAT on institutional computational resources. Thank you to Baylor College of Medicine Center for Advanced Magnetic Resonance Imaging (CAMRI) for use of imaging facility; including accommodations appropriate for families with young children.

Conflicts of Interest: The authors declare no conflicts of interest.

References

1. Foster-Cohen, S.; Edgin, J.O.; Champion, P.R.; Woodward, L.J. Early delayed language development in very preterm infants: Evidence from the MacArthur-Bates CDI. *J. Child Lang.* **2007**, *34*, 655–675. [CrossRef]
2. Gerstein, E.D.; Woodman, A.C.; Burnson, C.; Cheng, E.R.; Poehlmann-Tynan, J. Trajectories of externalizing and internalizing behaviors in preterm children admitted to a neonatal intensive care unit. *J. Pediatr.* **2017**, *187*, 111–118. [CrossRef] [PubMed]
3. Janssens, A.; Uvin, K.; Van Impe, H.; Laroche, S.M.F.; Van Reempts, P.; Deboutte, D. Psychopathology among preterm infants using the Diagnostic Classification Zero to Three. *Acta Paediatr.* **2009**, *98*, 1988–1993. [CrossRef] [PubMed]

4. Taylor, H.G.; Clark, C.A. Executive function in children born preterm: Risk factors and implications for outcome. *Semin. Perinatol.* **2016**, *40*, 520–529. [CrossRef] [PubMed]
5. Bouyssi-Kobar, M.; du Plessis, A.J.; McCarter, R.; Brossard-Racine, M.; Murnick, J.; Tinkleman, L.; Robertson, R.L.; Limperopoulos, C. Third trimester brain growth in preterm infants compared with in utero healthy fetuses. *Pediatrics* **2016**, *138*, e20161640. [CrossRef] [PubMed]
6. Kapellou, O.; Counsell, S.J.; Kennea, N.; Dyet, L.; Saeed, N.; Stark, J.; Maalouf, E.; Duggan, P.; Ajayi-Obe, M.; Hajnal, J.; et al. Abnormal cortical development after premature birth shown by altered allometric scaling of brain growth. *PLoS Med.* **2006**, *3*, e265. [CrossRef] [PubMed]
7. Nam, K.W.; Castellanos, N.; Simmons, A.; Froudist-Walsh, S.; Allin, M.P.; Walshe, M.; Murray, R.M.; Evans, A.; Muehlboeck, J.S.; Nosarti, C. Alterations in cortical thickness development in preterm-born individuals: Implications for high-order cognitive functions. *NeuroImage* **2015**, *115*, 64–75. [CrossRef]
8. Volpe, J.J. Brain injury in premature infants: A complex amalgam of destructive and developmental disturbances. *Lancet Neurol.* **2009**, *8*, 110–124. [CrossRef]
9. Volpe, J.J. The encephalopathy of prematurity—Brain injury and impaired brain development inextricably intertwined. *Semin. Pediatr. Neurol.* **2009**, *16*, 167–178. [CrossRef]
10. Gerstein, E.D.; Poehlmann-Tynan, J. Transactional processes in children born preterm: Influences of mother–child interactions and parenting stress. *J. Fam. Psychol.* **2015**, *29*, 777. [CrossRef]
11. Subedi, D.; DeBoer, M.D.; Scharf, R.J. Developmental trajectories in children with prolonged NICU stays. *Arch. Dis. Child.* **2016**, *102*, 29–34. [CrossRef]
12. Belfort, M.B.; Ramel, S.E. NICU Diet, Physical Growth and Nutrient Accretion, and Preterm Infant Brain Development. *Neoreviews* **2019**, *20*, e385–e396. [CrossRef]
13. Landry, S.H.; Smith, K.E.; Miller-Loncar, C.L.; Swank, P.R. Predicting cognitive-language and social growth curves from early maternal behaviors in children at varying degrees of biological risk. *Dev. Psychol.* **1997**, *33*, 1040. [CrossRef]
14. Steelman, L.M.; Assel, M.A.; Swank, P.R.; Smith, K.E.; Landry, S.H. Early maternal warm responsiveness as a predictor of child social skills: Direct and indirect paths of influence over time. *J. Appl. Dev. Psychol.* **2002**, *23*, 135–156. [CrossRef]
15. Kok, R.; Thijssen, S.; Bakermans-Kranenburg, M.J.; Jaddoe, V.W.; Verhulst, F.C.; White, T.; van IJzendoorn, M.H.; Tiemeier, H. Normal variation in early parental sensitivity predicts child structural brain development. *J. Am. Acad. Child Adolesc. Psychiatry* **2015**, *54*, 824–831. [CrossRef] [PubMed]
16. Thijssen, S.; Muetzel, R.L.; Bakermans-Kranenburg, M.J.; Jaddoe, V.W.; Tiemeier, H.; Verhulst, F.C.; White, T.; Van Ijzendoorn, M.H. H. Insensitive parenting may accelerate the development of the amygdala–medial prefrontal cortex circuit. *Dev. Psychopathol.* **2017**, *29*, 505–518. [CrossRef] [PubMed]
17. Keen, R. The development of problem solving in young children: A critical cognitive skill. *Annu. Rev. Psychol.* **2011**, *62*, 1–21. [CrossRef] [PubMed]
18. Gagne, J.R.; Liew, J.; Nwadinobi, O.K. How does the broader construct of self-regulation relate to emotion regulation in young children? *Dev. Rev.* **2021**, *60*, 100965. [CrossRef]
19. Blair, C.; Zelazo, P.D.; Greenberg, M.T. The Measurement of executive function in early childhood. *Dev. Neuropsychol.* **2005**, *28*, 561–571. [CrossRef] [PubMed]
20. Braun, K. The prefrontal-limbic system: Development, neuroanatomy, function, and implications for socioemotional development. *Clin. Perinatol.* **2011**, *38*, 685–702. [CrossRef] [PubMed]
21. Best, J.R.; Miller, P.H.; Naglieri, J.A. Relations between executive function and academic achievement from ages 5 to 17 in a large, representative national sample. *Learn. Individ. Differ.* **2011**, *21*, 327–336. [CrossRef]
22. Clark, C.A.; Woodward, L.J. Relation of perinatal risk and early parenting to executive control at the transition to school. *Dev. Sci.* **2015**, *18*, 525–542. [CrossRef] [PubMed]
23. Johnson, S.; Wolke, D.; Hennessy, E.; Marlow, N. Educational outcomes in extremely preterm children: Neuropsychological correlates and predictors of attainment. *Dev. Neuropsychol.* **2011**, *36*, 74–95. [CrossRef] [PubMed]
24. Dimitrova, R.; Pietsch, M.; Ciarrusta, J.; Fitzgibbon, S.P.; Williams, L.Z.J.; Christiaens, D.; Cordero-Grande, L.; Batalle, D.; Makropoulos, A.; Schuh, A.; et al. Preterm birth alters the development of cortical microstructure and morphology at term-equivalent age. *NeuroImage* **2021**, *243*, 118488. [CrossRef] [PubMed]
25. Tsujimoto, S. The Prefrontal Cortex: Functional Neural Development During Early Childhood. *Neuroscientist* **2008**, *14*, 345–358. [CrossRef] [PubMed]
26. Belsky, J.; De Haan, M. Annual research review: Parenting and children's brain development: The end of the beginning. *J. Child Psychol. Psychiatry* **2011**, *52*, 409–428. [CrossRef] [PubMed]
27. DeMaster, D.; Bick, J.; Johnson, U.; Montroy, J.J.; Landry, S.; Duncan, A.F. Nurturing the preterm infant brain: Leveraging neuroplasticity to improve neurobehavioral outcomes. *Pediatr. Res.* **2019**, *85*, 166–175. [CrossRef] [PubMed]
28. Duerden, E.G.; Card, D.; Lax, I.D.; Donner, E.J.; Taylor, M.J. Alterations in frontostriatal pathways in children born very preterm. *Dev. Med. Child Neurol.* **2013**, *55*, 952–958. [CrossRef]
29. Hodel, A.S. Rapid infant prefrontal cortex development and sensitivity to early environmental experience. *Dev. Rev.* **2018**, *48*, 113–144. [CrossRef]

30. Landry, S.H. The role of parents in early childhood learning. In *Encyclopedia on Early Childhood Development*; CEECD: Montreal, QC, Canada, 2008; pp. 1–6.
31. Luby, J.L.; Belden, A.; Harms, M.P.; Tillman, R.; Barch, D.M. Preschool is a sensitive period for the influence of maternal support on the trajectory of hippocampal development. *Proc. Natl. Acad. Sci. USA* **2016**, *113*, 5742–5747. [CrossRef]
32. Treyvaud, K.; Thompson, D.K.; Kelly, C.E.; Loh, W.Y.; Inder, T.E.; Cheong, J.L.Y.; Doyle, L.W.; Anderson, P.J. Early parenting is associated with the developing brains of children born very preterm. *Clin. Neuropsychol.* **2021**, *35*, 885–903. [CrossRef]
33. Vaughn, K.A.; Moore, B.D.; DeMaster, D. Nurturing the developing brain to reduce neurological delay. In *Diagnosis, Management and Modeling of Neurodevelopmental Disorders: The Neuroscience of Development*; Academic Press: Cambridge, MA, USA, 2021; pp. 471–480.
34. Eisenberg, N.; Cumberland, A.; Spinrad, T.L. Parental Socialization of Emotion. *Psychol. Inq.* **1998**, *9*, 241–273. [CrossRef]
35. Eisenberg, N.; Spinrad, T.L.; Eggum, N.D. Emotion-related self-regulation and its relation to children's maladjustment. *Annu. Rev. Clin. Psychol.* **2010**, *6*, 495–525. [CrossRef] [PubMed]
36. Landry, S.H.; Smith, K.E.; Swank, P.R. Responsive parenting: Establishing early foundations for social, communication, and independent problem-solving skills. *Dev. Psychol.* **2006**, *42*, 627. [CrossRef] [PubMed]
37. Morris, A.S.; Silk, J.S.; Steinberg, L.; Myers, S.S.; Robinson, L.R. The role of the family context in the development of emotion regulation. *Soc. Dev.* **2007**, *16*, 361–388. [CrossRef] [PubMed]
38. Pineda, R.G.; Neil, J.; Dierker, D.; Smyser, C.D.; Wallendorf, M.; Kidokoro, H.; Reynolds, L.C.; Walker, S.; Rogers, C.; Mathur, A.M.; et al. Alterations in brain structure and neurodevelopmental outcome in preterm infants hospitalized in different neonatal intensive care unit environments. *J. Pediatr.* **2014**, *164*, 52–60. [CrossRef] [PubMed]
39. Matas, L.; Arend, R.A.; Sroufe, L.A. Continuity of adaptation in the second year: The relationship between quality of attachment and later competence. In *Thebeginning. Readings on Infancy*; Columbia University Press: New York, NY, USA, 1978; pp. 547–556. [CrossRef]
40. Nordell, A.; Lundh, M.; Horsch, S.; Hallberg, B.; Aden, U.; Nordell, B.; Blennow, M. The acoustic hood: A patient-independent device improving acoustic noise protection during neonatal magnetic resonance imaging. *Acta Paediatr.* **2009**, *98*, 1278–1283. [CrossRef] [PubMed]
41. Li, G.; Nie, J.; Wang, L.; Shi, F.; Gilmore, J.H.; Lin, W.; Shen, D. Measuring the dynamic longitudinal cortex development in infants by reconstruction of temporally consistent cortical surfaces. *Neuroimage* **2014**, *90*, 266–279. [CrossRef] [PubMed]
42. Li, G.; Wang, L.; Shi, F.; Gilmore, J.H.; Lin, W.; Shen, D. Construction of 4D high-definition cortical surface atlases of infants: Methods and applications. *Med. Image Anal.* **2015**, *25*, 22–36. [CrossRef]
43. Li, G.; Wang, L.; Yap, P.T.; Wang, F.; Wu, Z.; Meng, Y.; Dong, P.; Kim, J.; Shi, F.; Rekik, I.; et al. Computational neuroanatomy of baby brains: A review. *NeuroImage* **2019**, *185*, 906–925. [CrossRef]
44. Wang, L.; Li, G.; Shi, F.; Cao, X.; Lian, C.; Nie, D.; Liu, M.; Zhang, H.; Li, G.; Wu, Z.; et al. Volume-based analysis of 6-month-old infant brain MRI for autism biomarker identification and early diagnosis. In Proceedings of the 21st International Conference on Medical Image Computing and Computer Assisted Intervention, Granada, Spain, 16–20 September 2018; Springer International Publishing: Cham, Switzerland, 2018; pp. 411–419. [CrossRef]
45. Wang, L.; Wu, Z.; Chen, L.; Sun, Y.; Lin, W.; Li, G. iBEAT V2. 0: A multisite-applicable, deep learning-based pipeline for infant cerebral cortical surface reconstruction. *Nat. Protoc.* **2023**, *18*, 1488–1509. [CrossRef] [PubMed]
46. Chen, L.; Wu, Z.; Hu, D.; Wang, Y.; Zhao, F.; Zhong, T.; Lin, W.; Wang, L.; Li, G. A 4D Infant Brain Volumetric Atlas based on the UNC/UMN Baby Connectome Project (BCP) Cohort. *NeuroImage* **2022**, *253*, 119097. [CrossRef]
47. Faul, F.; Erdfelder, E.; Buchner, A.; Lang, A.G. Statistical power analyses using G* Power 3.1: Tests for correlation and regression analyses. *Behav. Res. Methods* **2009**, *41*, 1149–1160. [CrossRef]
48. IBM Corp. *IBM SPSS Statistics for Windows*, version 27.0; IBM Corp: Armonk, NY, USA, 2020.
49. Topçiu, M.; Myftiu, J. Vygotsky theory on social interaction and its influence on the development of pre-school children. *Eur. J. Soc. Sci. Educ. Res.* **2015**, *2*, 172–179. [CrossRef]
50. Mermelshtine, R. Parent–child learning interactions: A review of the literature on scaffolding. *Br. J. Educ. Psychol.* **2017**, *87*, 241–254. [CrossRef] [PubMed]
51. Turnbull, O.H.; Salas, C.E. The neuropsychology of emotion and emotion regulation: The role of laterality and hierarchy. *Brain Sci.* **2021**, *11*, 1075. [CrossRef] [PubMed]
52. Belsky, J.; Pluess, M. Differential susceptibility to long-term effects of quality of child care on externalizing behavior in adolescence? *Int. J. Behav. Dev.* **2012**, *36*, 2–10. [CrossRef]

MDPI AG
Grosspeteranlage 5
4052 Basel
Switzerland
Tel.: +41 61 683 77 34

Children Editorial Office
E-mail: children@mdpi.com
www.mdpi.com/journal/children

www.ingramcontent.com/pod-product-compliance
Lightning Source LLC
Chambersburg PA
CBHW041524270926
51850CB00023BA/2634
* 9 7 8 3 7 2 5 8 4 2 6 1 2 *